Jack Hanford, ThD

Bioethics from a Faith Perspective
Ethics in Health Care for the Twenty-First Century

Pre-publication
REVIEWS,
COMMENTARIES,
EVALUATIONS . . .

"In *Bioethics from a Faith Perspective,* Dr. Jack Hanford provides a descriptive account of the issues to be found in biomedical research and practice. Because of his stance as a practitioner of a particular faith community, he has found it helpful to relate biomedical ethics to a faith perspective. Also, because of his concerns to deal with both reasoning and the relationship between ethical and faith issues, he has provided a thorough description of the works by Kohlberg, Rest, and Fowler in the development of fields of moral reasoning and faith development. Hanford's descriptions are accurate and presented in a form that will be understandable to the average college student or lay reader.

Dr. Hanford applies the framework from such a faith perspective to current issues in health care. He directly inquires as to the ethical issues involved in the use of transplants, the relationship between mental health and managed care, and the Human Genome Project. He provides specific references to the elderly and to bioethics issues for pastors and nurses.

In addition, Hanford offers biblical references for further discussion so that the book itself will be of very practical use to instructors in the fields of ethics, bioethics, medical research, and medical practice."

Clarence H. Snelling Jr., PhD
Professor Emeritus,
Iliff School of Theology,
Denver, Colorado

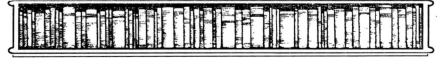

More pre-publication
REVIEWS, COMMENTARIES, EVALUATIONS . . .

"Dr. Hanford's book *Bioethics from a Faith Perspective* is the culmination of thirty years devotion to the field of bioethics. The book's rigorous intellectual appraisal of the field is typical of Dr. Hanford's approach to all areas of philosophical inquiry.

The reader is provided with insights into the part that faith plays in bioethical decision making. Yet, Dr. Hanford also insists upon the use of reason as a guide to the making of decisions.

Dr. Hanford takes an approach to his subject that is comprehensive and profound. He incorporates and analyzes in his examination of bioethics the 'interaction between moral philosophy, psychology, and theology. . . .'

Ultimately, Dr. Hanford provides the reader with a structure for understanding the importance in bioethical thinking and decision making of 'reason, logic, moral philosophy, and theology.' Dr. Hanford concludes, 'Faith perspective did and will make a difference.'

Dr. Hanford is now a mentor for the thousands."

Herbert L. Carson, PhD
Professor Emeritus of Humanities,
Ferris State University,
Big Rapids, MI

The Haworth Pastoral Press®
An Imprint of The Haworth Press, Inc.
New York • London • Oxford

Bioethics from a Faith Perspective

Ethics in Health Care for the Twenty-First Century

Bioethics from a Faith Perspective
Ethics in Health Care for the Twenty-First Century

Jack Hanford, ThD

The Haworth Pastoral Press®
An Imprint of The Haworth Press, Inc.
New York • London • Oxford

Published by

The Haworth Pastoral Press®, an imprint of The Haworth Press, Inc., 10 Alice Street, Binghamton, NY 13904–1580.

Portions of this book were taken from articles previously published by Human Sciences Press, Inc.:

Jack Hanford (1993). "Is the Faith of Faith Development Christian Faith?," *Journal of Pastoral Psychology, 42*(2), 95-105.
Jack Hanford (1993). "Religion, Medical Ethics, and Transplants," *Journal of Medical Humanities, 14*(1), 33-38.
Jack Hanford (1998). "Mental Health and Managed Care," *Journal of Religion and Health, 37*(2), 159-166.
Jack Hanford (2000). "A Public Religion and Biomedical Ethics," *Journal of Pastoral Psychology, 48*(3), 191-195.

Portions of this book were taken from an article published by the Christian Association for Psychological Studies:

Jack Hanford (1991). "The Relationship Between Faith Development of James Fowler and Moral Development of Lawrence Kohlberg: A Theoretical Review," *Journal of Psychology and Christianity, 10*(4), 306-310.

Cover design by Marylouise E. Doyle.

Library of Congress Cataloging-in-Publication Data

Hanford, Jack Tyrus.
    Bioethics from a faith perspective : ethics in health care for the twenty-first century / Jack Hanford
       p. cm.
    Includes bibliographical references and index.
    ISBN 0-7890-1509-9 (alk. paper)—ISBN 0-7890-1510-2 (alk. paper)
      1. Medical ethics—Religious aspects—Christianity. 2. Bioethics—Religious aspects—Christianity. I. Title.

R725.56 .H36 2002
174'.2—dc21
                                                   2001024392

CONTENTS

ABOUT THE AUTHOR

Jack Hanford, MDiv, MA, ThD, is Professor Emeritus of Biomedical Ethics at Ferris State University in Michigan. He has published articles in professional publications such as *Religious Education,* the *Journal for the Scientific Study of Religion, Media Development,* the *Western Journal of Speech Communication,* the *Journal of Psychology and Christianity,* the *Journal of Medical Humanities,* and the *Journal of Pastoral Psychology.* Dr. Hanford is a fellow of the Society for the Scientific Study of Religion, and a member of the American Philosophical Association, the American Academy of Religion, the Christian Association for Psychological Studies, the Society for Christian Ethics, and the Association of Moral Education. He is also an associate of the Hastings Center (the foremost center for biomedical ethics), The American Society of Bioethics and Humanities, the Center for Bioethics and Human Dignity and the Kennedy Institute of Ethics, as well as several other ethical and professional societies.

Foreword

Jack Hanford's very readable book joins a body of literature that examines the importance of faith perspectives as they influence the beliefs and values that persons bring to the experiences of health and disease, health care, and bioethics. Patients and families, doctors and nurses, pastors and friends all bring to the crises of health and illness formative and salient values, not only for health care decisions but also for general dispositions of suffering, hope, and courage.

In the great challenges of birth and death, pain and surgery, risk and resignation, these faith precepts bear far greater currency than economic, legal, or philosophical values. How we translate these parochial goods and evils (derivative of faith traditions) into public values, principles that can animate careful and respectful decisions in health care settings, is a great challenge of our time. We know that issues such as abortion and euthanasia, in vitro fertilization and transplantation are fraught with profound dimensions and gravity, yet we shrink from appropriation. Hanford's book is a handmaiden to this birth of faith-based bioethics.

Kenneth L. Vaux
Professor of Theological Ethics
Garrett Evangelical Theological Seminary

Preface

I have taught bioethics with university students, adults in churches, and many other places and have researched and published articles on bioethics for more than thirty years. These experiences have convinced me of the need for bioethics to be interpreted from a faith perspective. This book is the result of this teaching and research in bioethics, which also parallels the recent history of bioethics from 1970 to the twenty-first century. I participated in the very first meeting to develop bioethics, which was attended by philosophers, physicians, and theologians in Galveston, Texas. There, Edmund Pellegrino, Stephen Toulmin, H. Tristram Englehardt, and many others provided the leadership and scholarship to begin shaping a new field that had neither textbooks nor courses. Also, I met Howard Brody there, who was a medical and philosophy student at Michigan State University at that time in the early 1970s. Later in 1976, he wrote the first textbook, *Ethical Decisions in Medicine,* by a physician for physicians. I used this text and along with my students evaluated it. Brody acknowledged our contribution to the second edition in 1981. To continue my preparation, I spent three sabbaticals, culminating as a visiting professor, at the Medical Humanities Program of Michigan State University.

Also, I was taught bioethics at the Hastings Center by such luminaries as Daniel Callahan, Robert Veatch, and James Childress in at least six workshops beginning in 1975. During the summer of 1975, I continued learning moral and faith development with Lawrence Kohlberg, Carol Gilligan, Ann Colby, and Dan Candee at Harvard. In March 1989, I continued this work further by focusing on faith development in a research consultation with James Fowler, Karen DeNicola, and John Snarey at Emory University.

The National Endowment for the Humanities (NEH) supported my training through their summer seminars and institutes. In the summer of 1981 at Case Western Reserve University in Cleveland, I studied the distinctive problems of old age with Professor David Van Tassel and a practicing and teaching physician for the elderly, Joe

Foley. During the summer of 1983 at the University of Kentucky, I worked with Edmund Pellegrino, MD, and David Thomasma, PhD and have continued to keep up with them by reading most of what they have written. They stimulated and influenced much of my thinking in the philosophy and theology of medicine. Throughout the summer of 1987, I was a visiting fellow at Princeton University studying Christian ethics with Paul Sigmund, Paul Ramsey, and Stephen Post. Also, NEH funded me during the summer of 1994 at Iowa State University to write a research paper on ethics for medical technology from the history of technology. Much substance and criticism of most of my chapters came from work with these experts and colleagues, and I am grateful. But, of course, no one except the author is responsible for the interpretation of this book.

I am most grateful to my wife, Marilyn Brackett Hanford, for her work and support on this project and many other such challenges too numerous to list.

*   *   *

Writing a book requires many talents. I am profoundly grateful to Denise Moulter of Ferris State University for her computer expertise and editorial assistance. David C. Meyer of Meyer Publishing Enterprises functioned and helped as a consultant yet is most important as a friend for many years.

Introduction

The purpose for *Bioethics from a Faith Perspective* is to show the relevance, significance, and guidance that a faith perspective can offer for dealing with bioethical issues. This purpose stems from the fact that most Americans state their moral positions from the background of their faith traditions. Yet, some of these Americans might not have had opportunity to study the relation between their faith perspective and the difficult issues facing them in pursuing health care. This book makes visible a faith perspective functioning in health care discussions, which can have many uses for those Americans, students, and professionals in religion, medicine, and health care.

This purpose is expressed further in the following specific objectives for biomedical ethics from a faith perspective and for you, the reader.

1. First I distinguish and describe the relation between technical and ethical aspects of a health-related issue, problem, case, and decision, especially in the introduction, Chapter 9, and the conclusion.
2. I provide a framework of moral principles, theories, values, and faith viewpoints in order to construct critical positions on bioethical problems, cases, and policies in the introduction and Chapters 1, 2, and 3.
3. I name defining characteristics of a moral professional-client relationship related to faith in Chapters 1, 2, 3, 4, 6, 7, and 9 through 12.
4. I discern when medical ethics and faith commitments are therapeutic and when they are not in Chapters 4, 6, 7, and 9 through 12.
5. I describe a moral problem, a faith perspective, and a justified position on the problem within a health-related case and policy issue in each chapter from Chapter 5 to the conclusion.

THE TECHNICAL-ETHICAL DISTINCTION

If nonphysicians dare to approach biomedical ethics, we must understand the technical-ethical distinction first of all. Otherwise, most Americans and many doctors will assume that medical ethics includes vital issues to be decided exclusively by the physician. Along with most other bioethicists, I offer a division of labor between scholars in bioethics and physicians by presenting and clarifying throughout the book the technical-ethical distinction. Our realm of work and authority is within the ethical, which includes moral philosophy, religious convictions, the imperative of informed consent, the relation of the moral and the legal, justice and fairness issues such as allocation of scarce resources, and many other such moral issues. We also need at least a lay knowledge of the technical, but that is the realm of authority of physicians, many of whom also have much knowledge, but not exclusive knowledge, of ethics. In fact, physicians might have conflicts of interest in relation to ethical issues. Their authority is within the technical work of diagnosis, prognosis, treatments, side effects, and many other such technical matters. In the best of worlds, these two professions can work cooperatively yet independently, each recognizing the expertise of the other. This distinction can usually be made in practice and in deliberation of the decision-making process within bioethics, which must also be defined.

The term "bioethics" is the original, shortest, and broadest; "medical ethics" is the most narrow, often referring to the ethics of physicians. Thus, I prefer a middle term, "biomedical ethics." But these terms are often used interchangeably.

From the very beginning of the emergence of bioethics in the 1960s, Paul Ramsey insisted on the technical-ethical distinction, which gradually resulted in the physician's authority being somewhat limited to the technical or medical and allowed outsiders such as theologians, philosophers, attorneys, and others to enter debates with physicians and the public by asserting the authority of the ethical. This authority could be reinforced by legal and eventually Constitutional sanction. Without this technical-ethical distinction, all "ethical" problems could be reduced to "medical" problems, and there would be no bioethics as we now know it. Bioethics would be left exclusively to physicians, as Dr. Jack Kevorkian would prefer. Instead, bioethics as a part of ethics and/or theology is a process of thinking with care, moral principles, and a faith perspective about health care.

PROVIDE A FRAMEWORK

So, how does a faith perspective actually shed light on making a decision and taking an action on an issue in bioethics? We do decide and act from our beliefs, which have both cognitive and emotional meaning for us. I can also combine moral principles such as the bioethics mantra of beneficence, autonomy, and justice with a faith perspective, which adds agape, truth, freedom, and justice, especially for the oppressed. A faith perspective can add profound meaning to the principles of beneficence, autonomy, and justice. In this process of interaction between moral philosophy, psychology, and theology a meaningful framework can be created, providing a Christian perspective broadly and inclusively defined. (Other religious traditions also, of course, provide faith perspectives.) The Christian perspective, which is the one I know best, can illuminate and guide decisions and policies in health care. Therefore, this faith needs to be dealt with, although the diversity of faith traditions in America means that we have difficulty dealing with religion and faith. Because of this difficult problem, I studied and am guided by scholars such as James Fowler, Edmund Pellegrino, Ian Barbour (1993), and others who focus on health care and its technology through the lens of a Christian faith perspective.

This purpose and faith perspective need to be viewed within a period of history from 1880 to 2000 and within the more recent emergence of bioethics (1960-2000). During this period of history, the prestige of science escalated while religion declined, and medicine rode the back of science while religion was perceived to be in conflict with science, even involved in warfare with science. Powerful authority for the physician came from the rigor of medical education based on science plus the genius and power of the American Medical Association (discussed further in Chapter 9). But by the 1960s, almost all authority, including professional, was called into question.

Thus, while many authority structures and institutions in America were being challenged, if not destroyed, during the 1960s, a new structure in the form of bioethics was being created. Although no single intent or influence created the new field of study, we can explore several contributing influences. At least two theologians produced ideas and literature to influence this new movement. Joseph Fletcher (1954) wrote *Morals and Medicine* from his early deontological perspective, meaning that principles decide what is right. Paul Ramsey, who disagreed with Fletcher, nevertheless assisted the publication of Fletcher's book by Princeton University, where Ramsey was a professor. Later, Ramsey (1970) published his own seminal book, *The Patient As Person,* one of the famous Beecher lectures at Yale. These sources contributed to a major change in attitudes toward health care by Americans from the 1960s into the 1970s and beyond. Fletcher's insistence on personal rights and later on situational ethics were used to challenge traditional authority, including that of physicians. Such challenges exposed the lack of an adequate basis for trust, which led to and exposed a general erosion of trust. Also, Ramsey expressed outrage, especially toward abuses of consent in research on children, incompetents, and the lack of care for dying patients.

The most important change in the history of bioethics in recent decades has been the secularization of the field. Although theologians such as Fletcher and Ramsey and others provided some of the original source and stimulation for the emergence of the field, there has not yet been a significant public expression of religion in bioethics. Daniel Callahan (1990) has provided his personal experience as an illustration of this secularization of bioethics and the exclusion of religion from the field. When Callahan first explored bioethics in the mid-1960s, the only resources available were theological, especially Catholic, and the tradition of medicine itself, which had been strongly influenced by religion. The public expression of the Roman Catholic Church on procreation and population issues in the 1960s presented problems to Callahan. More specifically, the conservative turn of Catholicism away from Vatican II influenced Callahan to turn toward the secular for resources for dealing with bioethics, especially on abortion, reproductive issues, and population control. Because he became convinced that he could not work effectively through the Church, he established his secular and prestigious think-tank on bioethics, the Hastings Center.

Since Callahan turned away from the private and personal significance of religion, he also set aside the significance of religion in the public and collective realm of biomedicine. This move facilitated his communication with secular institutions. But at the same time, Callahan identified three results of this disappearance or denaturing of religion from public discourse: we are left too dependent on the law as a source of morality, we are bereft of particular moral communities, and we are also bereft of wisdom from religious traditions. Although Callahan is a part of the exclusion of religion, he also paradoxically notes the need for the inclusion of a public religion within biomedical ethics (used here interchangeably with bioethics).

While bioethics expanded into public recognition from 1960 to the present, the religion of its beginnings seemed to almost disappear into a private closet. The field of biomedical ethics was taken over during recent decades by the secular forces of medicine, academia, law, the media, and most recently by economics and health policy. For example, a philosopher with the University of Alabama School of Medicine, Gregory Pence (1990), wrote a text, *Classic Cases in Medical Ethics: Accounts of the Cases That Have Shaped Medical Ethics with Philosophical, Legal, and Historical Backgrounds.* Not only is there no mention of religion in this title, but the subject index lists only four obscure references under religion. In a similar way, religion is conspicuous by its absence in most of the medical ethics texts I have reviewed over thirty years.

Mark Siegler (1991), a distinguished physician, and others suggest a clear vision of the right place for religion in biomedical ethics, the view that private religion should be integrated into public life. As Parker Palmer (1981) also concludes, "The very health of the private realm depends on the health of the public sphere" (p. 31). Religion can make a forceful public expression and potentially help create a more civil society.

For the future, I offer a rationale and program for the public expression of faith (especially in Chapter 5) in a civil medical ethics. Specifically, the public church, synagogue, and other communities need to consider taking a public role. Theological support for this approach is offered in a dissertation by J. Tubbs (1990, p. 382), who concludes that all four of the theologians James Gustafson, Stanley Hauerwas, Richard McCormick, and Paul Ramsey appeal to the theological notion that our lives are gifts from God, which calls for a response of gratitude from Christians. The time is ripe now for a public faith to make its contribution to bioethics. This contribution can be distinctive to a biblical tradition, useful and pragmatic to bioethics, and enriching to American culture. For example, a public faith is especially important for organ donation, quality managed care, justice between generations, and the future development of biomedical ethics. There appears to be a consensus in the medical ethics literature that organ donation be achieved through volunteerism. Martin Marty (1990) notes "that two-thirds of American citizens' volunteer hours are attracted through organized religion" (p. 15). These two statements suggest that the public church is the institution of choice to carry out the task and meet the demand for organs.

The notion of the public church has caught the imagination of many religious leaders. Marty (1990) defines this theological conviction to include the Catholic Church, the mainline Protestant denominations, the evangelicals, and others. These Catholic and Protestant ecumenical groups and others could proceed by educating their individual congregations about the consensus mentioned earlier. Such education could then spread throughout the society. Since members of the congregation hopefully know and trust one another, the education would be sensitive to persons' needs and produce greater cooperation toward donating organs, interpreting quality care in managed care, and offering their faith perspective to bioethics for a good society.

America needs competent pastors, nurses, and physicians to provide guidance for the profound religious dimension of bioethics. Many of the bioethical issues are specifically religious. Abortion is an obvious example, along with playing God, prayer and healing, spirituality and evangelism, death and suicide, and the many cases involving Jehovah's Witnesses and Christian Scientists.

The book includes a description of a faith perspective in the first half and presents the perspective in practice in the second half. Specific objectives one through four are prevalent throughout the book. Objective five provides a focus for the second half of the book, dealing with issues in practice such as organ donation and managed care. But first, you are invited to join a building project to construct a rational framework for dealing with bioethics and its vital issues.

Chapter 1

Framework:
Advancing Moral Reasoning
Toward a Faith Perspective

In my thirty years of teaching bioethics, I have found that most students and others grasp the moral and faith stages readily. Some proceed to analyze, evaluate, and construct a meaningful framework coherent with Christian faith broadly and inclusively interpreted. Before reporting this teaching experience and research, I present a sketch of the moral stages of reasoning. They are not intended as a test for measuring personality. They are simply a description of the longitudinal progression of moral reasoning derived from Lawrence Kohlberg's interviews (1981, 1984) scrutinized by four decades of graduate students and other professional researchers. These stages are age-related, but they are not strictly determined by chronological age.

Within level I, the preconventional level, there are two stages, namely stages 1 and 2. Stage 1 is the punishment and obedience orientation, which is common for persons at the earliest ages, two to seven. Roughly, this is the thinking of a young child who does what he or she is told regardless of consequences. This reasoning operates to avoid punishment because of fear. Whether a child does or does not do what the parent says is a content decision that is what one decides. Kohlberg insists that this stage of reasoning is discerned by form, that is why one decides. Thus a young child might not do what the parent says because the child might be so thoroughly egocentric that he or she does not even consider the voice of the other.

Stage 2, instrumental relativism, requires additional assertion of feeling and thinking for his or her own interests and needs, roughly ages eight to fourteen. By instrumental relativism, I mean the instrumental satisfaction of needs. For example, a child who thinks about fair play emphasizes fair play that benefits or satisfies him or her in stage 2. According to Jean Piaget's work, at this stage the rules of the game are used and followed in order to play in the game. Cognitive reasoning later in life at this stage might mean, for example, doing a particular job because one gets paid regardless of what other considerations might be at stake. Taking a bribe might also illustrate this second stage of instrumental relativism and self-absorbed satisfaction.

Now we move from level I, preconventional moral judgments, to conventional level II moral judgments, which include stages 3 and 4. Stage 3 is characteristic of early teenagers' thinking and feeling. They are very much concerned about conforming with the group, which is what we mean by interpersonal concordances. In terms of early child development too, this conformity often suggests being nice to receive approval. For adults, stage 3 relies especially on a professional role that provides the authority to sanction decisions by health professionals and others. This moral reasoning might have important implications for the teacher-intern relationship and other such professional relationships. Interns need basic learning from the teacher, and the intern might simply copy the teacher's behavior.

Kohlberg believes most adult Americans reason in stage 4 when making basic ethical decisions. Stage 4 is the law and order orientation. Kohlberg believed that President Richard Nixon was operating in this particular stage by emphasizing the simple reasoning that most things are solved by black-and-white decisions sanctioned by the authority of institutions. Stage 4½, if Kohlberg is correct, is the stage of reasoning characteristic of most college students. This moral reasoning inherits certain traditional values but also questions these values. This reasoning includes the relative-absolute conflict. Personal relativism defines what is right by reference to the person such as it is right because the person said so. Kohlberg (1984, p. 438) defines an absolute claim as unquestionable because the claim is always right when it refers to a principle. There are no exceptions. Because this claim is logically vulnerable, Kohlberg does not affirm absolutes but he does affirm universals (in stage 6).

Next is level III, the postconventional, moving from stage 4 or 4½ to stage 5. If we carry over the earlier analogy of President Nixon's reasoning being in stage 4, then we might characterize stage 5 with principles that are built into our structures of government. These ideas in the Constitution made Nixon accountable to principles of justice beyond his own basic authority position.

Stage 5, the social contract legalistic orientation, emphasizes that decisions are based on principled moral judgment, principles such as those in the Declaration of Independence, that all people are accountable to the law and all are equal under the law. These principles enable one to move beyond the law and order orientation of stage 4 of the mass society. Here in stage 4 there is an emphasis on the legal, but stage 5 thinking trumps the general rules of society. Most moral reasoning is predominantly in stage 4 and fluctuates from stages 3 to 5. Cognitive development advances when stage 5 reasoning appeals to the person reasoning in stage 4.

Teachers and learners can facilitate their advancement from stage 4 to stage 5 and possibly also to stage 6. These stage 5 and 6 reasoners generally do not reach this degree of sophistication until they are in their thirties, roughly. They learn to reason with self-chosen universal ethical principles and faith convictions. They operate autonomously, freely from within themselves because they have internalized basic objective principles and faith perspectives that guide their conduct. This moral reasoning enables them to take full responsibility for their own lives and for concern about others. It uses universal reasons that go beyond society in order to imagine and do what is ethical. Such thinking might involve civil disobedience. For example, Kohlberg believed that Martin Luther King Jr., Mother Teresa, Mahatma Ghandi, Jesus, the Buddha, and others demonstrated stage 6 moral reasoning.

The stages and levels of moral reasoning are also useful for providing a roughly sketched framework for analyzing and evaluating distinctions between various relationships existing in health care. For example, a practitioner reasoning in stage 1 would try to avoid malpractice simply to avoid punishment, not out of concern for the patient. Stage 1 reasoning might also embrace extreme punishment in a sadistic sense such as against the patient or against the practitioner. The notion of the "meanest cut" imposed by a practitioner such as in malpractice might express this reasoning. As I noted earlier, stage 2 reasoning is characterized as instrumental in the sense of one person using another for his or her own benefit. For instance, a practitioner might relate to the client only for selfish compensation, thereby using the client to pay the bills of the clinic and to make profits. Stage 3 identifies the reasoning in parental relationships. This stance implies that the client is metaphorically a child, that is, a dependent and subordinate. Stage 4 reasoning is dominated by legal appeals as the decisive end of moral deliberation. In contrast, Kohlberg defines "moral" by appeal to rational, objective, universal principles such as autonomy, beneficence, and justice. This moral reasoning paves the way to stage 5, characterized by a mutually agreed contract such as the U.S. Constitution. This point of development of moral reasoning ends Kohlberg's definite stages, based on rigorous longitudinal research over forty years. But consistent with Kohlberg, we can hypothesize a much-needed stage 6 covenant relationship supported by James Fowler's (1981) stage 6 faith perspective. This rich biblical conviction points the direction for guidance toward a therapeutic bioethics, including the characteristics of a quality professional relationship as called for in objectives two and three (from the Introduction).

Kohlberg also uses the stages to analyze moral reasoning within and between institutions. His research shows much stage 2 thinking in prisons; much stage 3 thinking in schools, the military, and hospitals. His work was committed especially to the discovery of methods to advance moral reasoning in public schools.

In my earlier research (in Rest, 1986, pp. 63-64, 209), I produced and published a significant finding, namely, that it was possible to advance principled and logical moral reasoning with nursing students. The question for the study was: Will nursing students taking the bioethics course advance their moral reasoning (measured on the Defining Issues Test [DIT] and interviews) more than a comparable group of nursing students who did not take the course?

The DIT was given as a pretest and a posttest to sixteen persons in an experimental class and sixteen persons in a regular class (the control group). The data revealed that the average gain of 8.1 points was significant at the 0.01 level of confidence. Thus, moral reasoning was advanced significantly.

The DIT is derived from a substantial database, and its reliability and validity have been demonstrated by many different investigators. Researchers (Martin, Shafto, and Vandeinse, 1977) independent of James Rest have replicated some of his research and confirmed the reliability, validity, and design of the Defining Issues Test. From use of the test along with interviewing the same subjects, I believe it does measure moral reasoning.

Specifically, students who repeated very low DIT scores also showed on their final exams an inability to present and argue by using moral principles, and they had a commitment to ethical relativism (Kohlberg, 1981, pp. 2-7), that is, there are no objective moral claims but only subjectivism. In response to six essay questions asking for principled reasoning, these students responded that they could not decide reasons for or against transplants, genetic control, and euthanasia. Also, they asserted that others cannot decide or choose because no one has a right to decide, and if anyone did, he or she would be playing God. Thus the reference to "God" is actually in the form of a relativistic claim. If our orientation is relativist, we will interpret reasons as arbitrary and simply dependent on the reasoner. This thinking also came out in class.

Someone fixated in the conventional level (stages 3 and 4) will hesitate to consider both sides of a moral issue, because such consideration is viewed not as a rational process but as getting in the way of definite decisions. These students will press the teacher for answers and not be satisfied that level III, the postconventional (stages 5 and 6), provides a perspective on the issues rather than an answer (Boyd, 1976, p. 164).

In contrast, a student who scored high on the DIT could clearly write essays in which relativism was clearly defined, moral principles were identified and compared so the conflicts in principles could be reasoned through, and a deliberate and provisional decision was made for a principle or principles that adjudicate the conflict. This is an example of principled moral reasoning. Another high scorer asserts the importance of going beyond the arbitrary by identifying objective principles such as respect for life and coming to a definite position with reasoned backing or support. These examples suggest that persons scoring high on the DIT can do more than recognize principles, they can also consistently and coherently reason with principles, which is a significant task of production or creativity. These persons apply principles not only to themselves but especially to others, and argue for civil disobedience, going beyond the law by reasoning with justified moral and faith principles. These findings suggest that writing essay questions is effective for evaluation along with the use of the Defining Issues Test.

The students' responses on the evaluation suggest their appreciation for being encouraged to think, to perceive, and to sense the importance of being involved in a personal, psychological, and developmental process of learning. The teaching strategies of Socratic dialogue, discussion, existential personal involvement, and exploration of faith perspectives were evidently useful, helpful, and effective. The responses also show that a variety of teaching strategies are desirable. This finding is supported by other research. For example, from the Ontario Institute for Studies in Education, the Pickering Study by Beck (1972) shows that a variety of teaching strategies used over a year are effective in stimulating moral development.

My personal research and experience have been reinforced by additional massive research over thirty years showing that advanced moral reasoning correlates with competent practice. For example, research from T.J. Sheehan and colleagues (1980) to that of Self (1994) has shown that high scores on the Defining Issues Test predict good, superior clinical performance among physicians, nurses, dentists, and other health professionals.

Among the many very distinguished graduate students taught by Kohlberg, there appears to be a consensus that the late James Rest is still the dean of neo-Kohlbergian research. Rest (1999), in his most recent publication, shows with extensive data that this approach can meet the critics "head on" and still produce new findings attesting to its fruitfulness in shedding light on postconventional thinking on culture and bioethics.

Rest (1999) does not follow Kohlberg's commitment to form or abstract structures over content or specific cultural beliefs. Instead, Rest (1999) presents schema, that is a logically organized plan, vision, viewpoint, or perspective, which includes content and excludes form. Rest thereby separates his research from the many criticisms leveled at Kohlberg by psychologists, philosophers, and theologians that Kohlberg focused too exclusively on form. Kohlberg's concentration on form for reliability in empirical measurement tends to reduce morality to form and to exclude specific moral contents. Since he was determined to maintain a reliable or consistently empirical method, he removed content (i.e., *what* we decide) and thereby reduced morality to form (i.e., *why* we decide).

In my judgment, religious morality requires a particular content. Suppose we apply the exclusive concentration on form to an actual moral issue. Can we really settle for only attending to why we think abortion is moral or not? Isn't it obvious that *what* we think about abortion is crucial? Kohlberg seems to suggest that only structure develops and that content cannot be treated developmentally. But research shows that the content of medical ethics and moral philosophy stimulates moral reasoning. Separating form from content distorts moral judgment and seems contradictory to the natural law tradition which includes both content and form. Focusing exclusively on form makes morality too abstract. Kohlberg implicitly recognizes this, because he does not consistently stick to his emphasis on form in his own moral judgments. He makes content decisions on capital punishment, Watergate, My Lai massacre, etc.

Another important issue is what criteria to use for evaluating Kohlberg's work. The criteria Kohlberg himself employs come from the formalist tradition in philosophy, including thinkers such as I. Kant, D. D. Raphael, R. M. Hare, W. Frankena, and J. Rawls, and from the developmental psychology and epistemology of Piaget and Dewey. Kohlberg also adds the criteria of pragmatic results. His test is whether social psychological inquiry produces insight into philosophical problems, and his inquiry found a parallel relation between psychological and philosophical moral development. But the validity of this relation needs further study.

The Defining Issues Test scores represent expressions of schemas rather than stages or forms. The strength of a schema, such as the progressive versus orthodox positions or perspectives, is a stronger predictor of behavior than church affiliation. This point needs to be considered in evaluating Harold Koenig's (1999) research because he relies heavily on a measure of church affiliation and attendance, and I found no reference to "schema" in his index but he does use schematic representation.

Rest (1999) and his colleagues have produced much research that has provoked controversy and thereby stimulated more research which will continue into the future. Inevitably the controversy, even political and religious warfare, was triggered by the progressives and the orthodox. Specifically, the orthodox have charged that Rest's research is biased against them. For example, a colleague, J. Lawrence (1987), found that radical fundamentalist seminarians appeared stuck in stage or schema 4 even though their DIT scores showed that they could reason beyond schema 4. Rest (1999, p. 58) suggested that their reasoning was not being utilized in making moral judgments because they were putting their reasoning aside in favor of their biblical theology that God decided moral judgments. The seminarians relied on this authority rather than assert their own thinking. Rest's successor, Stephen Thoma, has created a device to measure the utilization of a schema, such as whether the seminarians utilized faith content but not reason. This controversy is producing more research now and will into the future. Such work is much needed because our history shows that fundamentalism has been a source of an anti-intellectual attitude in America.

We need to integrate the research by Rest, Fowler, and John Snarey on moral and faith thinking and on the culture wars between orthodoxy, stage 4 fundamentalism according to Rest (1999), and progressivism. Rest and Fowler accept European enlightenment thinking, which provides a common foundation. Also, Rest (1999, p. 68) identifies Reinhold Niebuhr (1943) and P. Tillich (1957) as postconventional in their reasoning.

Another recent thirty-year production of research especially important for this book was published by H. Everding and colleagues (1998). This summary of research presents cognitive development manifested in adult faith perspectives and viewpoints interpreting self-understanding, authority of the Bible, tradition, beliefs, empathy, justice, diversity, and community. This book is distinctive and useful for integrating such research on moral and faith development with bioethics.

For example, Everding and colleagues (1998, pp. 125-137) present four perspectives on faith roughly representing the reasoning of Fowler's faith stages 2 through 6. They use these distinctive perspectives to elucidate or expose four meanings of empathy. This is very important for bioethics because empathy is increasingly an essential concept for distinguishing four different qualities in a practitioner-patient relationship. Basic elements of the meaning of empathy were embedded within the thought and method of Kohlberg. Empathy requires the capacity and skill of role-taking in our relationships and in thinking rationally and emotionally about moral issues. For instance, men need to be able to imagine the position of women facing an unexpected pregnancy when men deal with the ethics of abortion. The challenge is to vicariously wear the shoes of the other. In debate, role-taking demands that we state the position of our opponent to his or her satisfaction. Empathy is necessary for advancing our ethical reasoning, which deals with the conflict in moral dilemmas, understanding the logic in the next stage or schema above our present thinking, and role-taking where the cognitive and affective meet and work together.

Health practitioners are increasingly insisting on empathy for effective practice. The presence of the empathic relationship facilitates healing and comforting. Perhaps even the placebo effect might be produced by such a relationship. The ultimate meaning of empathy in the Judeo-Christian tradition is in the incarnation of God in Jesus, who took on the suffering and death of the world to embody the hope and faith of the world. The substance of this faith perspective is needed for bioethics.

A faith perspective creates and provides the primary motivation for one's life. The faith that provides motivation to learn is from sources in the Jewish, Christian, and other religious traditions. These sources stimulate vision, courage, and critical insight for bioethics. In recent decades, faith has motivated conservatives and progressives toward a more academically sound approach to religion, education, and bioethics. We need to develop further an approach to teaching and learning that is academically sound and motivates inquiry into faith, ethics, and bioethics.

Such motivation is dependent on our beliefs, specifically our faith viewpoint. This faith creates through imagination the religious experience that stimulates motivation to learn, to change, to act, to become moral. Religious experience is the intrinsic motivation that provides the autonomy for the study of religion and commitment to ethics. This faith is intentional and requires an object that is sacred or numinous.

In 1960, 80 percent of students wanted meaning in their education. In 1980, only 40 percent wanted it, which shows a threatening trend. The inquiry about meaning is typically religious and therefore integral to a faith perspective. The meaning a task has for a person determines his or her motivation to perform the task, as in bioethics. Achievement motivation includes a desire or interest, i.e., a need to excel.

Although the philosophical principles of Kohlberg and Rest provide needed action guides for moral practice, the persons using these principles also might need the power of the faith perspective of Fowler to motivate moral practice in spite of the pressures of a commodified, commercial world. In fact, all of these research programs provide much promise for relating a faith perspective to bioethics. Thus, the specific content of the faith perspective must be clarified further in the following chapters.

Chapter 2

The Relationship Between Moral Development and Faith Development

We now move further toward a faith perspective, because faith can contribute to a rational comprehensive framework and provide motivation toward a therapeutic medical ethic (used interchangeably with bioethics). One representative example of such perspective comes from James Fowler, who originally created the rational and universal stages of faith along with Lawrence Kohlberg when both were at Harvard.

Positions on faith and bioethical issues require a framework for justification. The public needs to be persuaded with good reasons. I think Stanley Hauerwas (1997) justifies his claims even while he repudiates apologetics and reasons. His stories are nevertheless compelling and thereby produce justification. If correct, these points provide an understanding of why Hauerwas is one of our foremost public theologians, especially in terms of public impact, even while he also repudiates public theology such as that espoused by Ronald Thiemann (1996) of Harvard Divinity. The dialogue between these two theologians gives us clues as to how to present theology and ethics. Both have produced serious and profound insights from history and narrative although they embody different attitudes toward America, revelation, and liberalism. They can move us from a domesticated civil religion toward a prophetic theology. Within this process, rational justification is necessary but not sufficient for us to know when public religion enhances life and when it does not. To answer, our claims must be "publicly accessible," as emphasized by Kent Greenawalt (1988), Martin Marty (1991), and Ronald Thiemann (1996). To be accessible, claims must be justified by logic, science, and reason. Kohlberg and Fowler provide this kind of justification for our faith perspective.

Lawrence Kohlberg (1927-1987) was recognized as the leading researcher on moral development for much of the twentieth century. For him, the core definition of morality is justice, a rational and universal principle that functions to adjudicate conflict of rights. Although Kohlberg is interested in religion, he claims no expertise. Rather, he points to James Fowler to explicate the meaning of faith and its challenge to moral development and to justice.

Since the 1980s, there has been a major controversy over theory. Kohlberg (1974) claims that moral development precedes faith development. On the contrary, Fowler (1978) claims that faith development in stages 5 and 6 precedes moral development, because faith provides the motivation for advancing into these highest stages. Clarification of this sequencing of the stages will be made by delineating the nature and relationship of the constructs justice and faith.

Fowler and Kohlberg present independent yet related (parallel) stage models of human development. They have designed different theories, yet each has shown an interest in the ideas of the other. If the precise relationship between Kohlberg's moral development and Fowler's faith development could be known, this knowledge might shed light on the complex relation between morality and religion, which has stymied scholars for centuries.

In the early 1970s, some of Fowler's students at Harvard Divinity School began to investigate the relationship between Kohlberg's concept of morality and Fowler's concept of faith. One problem that presented itself and continues to surface is whether morality precedes faith development or whether faith is a prerequisite to moral development. Regardless of which precedes the other, research shows a strong parallel between moral stages and faith stages. Shulik (1979) reported a .75 correlation, and F. C. Power and Kohlberg (1980, p. 359) found the correlation to be .81. Nevertheless, the focus here is that Kohlberg claimed that faith need not precede moral development, although it is not unusual to find religious faith among those at the highest stages of moral development. By contrast, Fowler believed that faith is needed to provide the motivation for advancing to higher levels of moral understanding, and therefore faith is a necessary antecedent condition.

Before I proceed, basic concepts such as morality and justice, faith and religion must be clarified in order to pursue theoretical statements concerning faith and moral development. I turn first to Kohlberg's view of morality and justice and then to Fowler's definition of faith and religion.

KOHLBERG AND MORALITY

Kohlberg's (1982) central concept of morality is that of justice. He believed that philosophers of deontological and utilitarian persuasion are in general agreement on the principles of justice, and that the official basis of political morality in the United States is one in which justice and fairness are primary. Because philosophers are less apt to agree on what constitutes the good life than on a definition of morality, and because the U.S. Constitution allows for a variety of religious beliefs but not for a variety of interpretations of what the Constitution says, justice or fairness rather than faith or religion must be the cornerstone of what it means to be moral.

Kohlberg (1974) acknowledged from his interviews with children that talk about God provided content ranging from stage 1 to stage 5. Kohlberg understood this content (not form) as a nonmoral value and did not view "God," per se, as normative, but considered the principle of justice as normative for talk of God and other expressions of religion. Various expressions about "God" were evaluated by the standard of the stages of moral reasoning. Justice could be universal, but religion or faith could not be. He did, however, add a stage 7, a metaphor for the highest level of maturity, which includes the religious, moral, humanistic, and mystical ideas that help to explain the meaning of life and death, but he did not consider stage 7 to be a true moral stage that could be measured and understood like the other six stages. Stage 7 asks the ultimate question—why be moral? The answer transcends both cognitive and humanistic interpretation.

Kohlberg further separated advanced ideals of justice from the religious sphere when he wrote of Martin Luther King Jr., whom he greatly admired. Kohlberg (1974) wrote that "Martin Luther King spoke and educated not primarily as a minister of religion, not primarily as a spokesman of the welfare of Blacks, but as he [King] said 'as a drum major for justice'" (p. 10).

FOWLER AND FAITH

The concept of faith can be clarified from studying the works of James Fowler (1996), who is currently the major writer in the area of faith development in human personality. Fowler interprets faith as a verb, that is, "faithing" or searching for meaning. Faithing also functions to construct coherent world perspectives and is a way of knowing, valuing, and committing. This function of knowing and giving meaning also provides authority by way of reasoned conviction. Faith implies loyalty and fidelity; concrete symbols such as a cross or ring become meaningful representations of one's faith.

The meaning of faith can be sketched by a brief description of the six stages as they develop from infancy to late adulthood. The overall comprehensive image of this life cycle is a cone such as an ice cream cone. We grow from the bottom point toward the wide open vision of the top suggesting that life is not linear but dramatic, cyclical, with an open and promising future.

Fowler begins with infancy because of his intense interest in the early maturation and function of the brain. But the first stage is young childhood characterized in ages two to seven. Both Kohlberg and Fowler describe this form of thinking as cognitive egocentrism. For instance, this child might believe the sun and moon are following him or her. Their faith, meaning trust, is fused and dependent on others, especially the parents. This relationship shapes the youngster's feelings, thoughts, and images. Fantastic beliefs have no problem with facts. Parents typically provide the rudiments for representing God.

Stage two thinking is usually expressed in childhood during the years eight to thirteen. The assurance of faith is secure in concrete and literal cognitive and emotional structures of thought and stories. This faith and morality of Kohlberg's instrumental thinking are illustrated in the absolute conviction that God helps those who help themselves.

Stage three describes thinking through the teen years which embodies conventional faith based on conformity to parents and/or peers. The form of these beliefs will depend substantially on whether the capacity for abstract comprehension is functioning. Authority for faith is often decided by a group which might include a church or a gang. Such faith is mutual and interpersonal but not critically examined.

Stage four usually emerges during the twenties. Advancement in reasoning, however, is not as dependent on chronological age as much as it is on education. Faith in this time is especially reflective, it is still personal but thinking almost inevitably becomes critical. Faith might be dealt with by procedural knowing, that is, by the procedures or method of science or the due process of the judicial system. These methodologies might be used either to strengthen faith-seeking understanding or to threaten commitment to faith. Whether faith should be rigidly certain and closed or an ongoing open quest describes a struggle for faith during this period.

Stage five, during the thirties and beyond, is described as conjunctive faith. To be conjunctive requires integration, sometimes a union of convictions, and being thoroughly critical by being both positive and skeptical about faith. Religious thought and especially Christian thought are paradoxical. How is a young adult to accept paradoxes and still be logical? Faith at this point in life is not simple but complex and perhaps perplexing. Ought faith be lived in such tension or should it be comforting? These challenging questions call for openness, humility, and insight into symbols and metaphors.

Stage six provides the completion of a journey toward faith in mid and late life. This faith is universal. It must complete the work of the earlier stages, especially stage five. This process of faith requires openness, decisiveness, and tolerance. Such tolerance faces differences, is well grounded in wisdom, and strives toward universal inclusiveness in justice and love. Universal faith includes particular religious traditions, is authentic, and prays for saintliness through faithful change and transformation.

In constructing faith stages, Fowler (1978) wanted his students to develop an understanding of their own faith as well as to interpret theology as an expression of faith. To do this, Fowler (1974) used the faith stages to make qualitative distinctions between various theologies such as black theology, liberation theology, or a balanced theology. Fowler's emphasis on the cognitive function of faith as faith knowing included reason and therefore was not to be equated with mystical knowing. The faith stages also represented an expansion of consciousness, greater inclusiveness of persons, and more tolerance of others. Faith stages function as guidelines for thinking theologically and imagining the meaning of God as related to us in the world. Fowler's highest stage, stage 6 or universalizing faith, includes a commitment to the Kingdom of God, the unity of all persons, and the fulfillment of human rights and justice. Thus, faith at its highest level includes advancement in moral understanding.

Faith functions to create the motivation needed to pursue human rights and justice. An example of such faith, according to Fowler, is seen in the faith development of Malcolm X, who became increasingly concerned about human dignity and liberation and sought social and economic justice. Malcolm X was empowered by anger, from experiences of the humiliation of his father, mother, and people. The rage that resulted influenced Malcolm's identity and shaped him as a leader for a liberation movement against oppression. His negative identity as "Satan" functioned to name him as a prophet, especially against the religion that sanctioned oppression. The humiliation of attending segregated schools made his cynicism logical and almost appropriate to his view of the world. While in prison, his faith further motivated him to become a leader for the liberation of black Muslims.

Although one may question Malcolm X's right to advocate violence, separatism and intolerance, Fowler deals with the matter more from the perspective of faith than from the perspective of moral behavior. Fowler sees Malcolm's faith as in transition from stage 4 faith to stage 5 faith. First, Fowler (1974) defines stage 4 as individuating-reflexive:

> It provided clear, sharp boundaries of inclusion and exclusion, it dichotomized the world into the saved and the damned; it provided ethical guidelines that required discipline and self-sacrifice; and it demanded total subordination of individual will and autonomy to the authority of Allah. (p. 16)

Thus Malcolm was characterized as a "totalizer" at stage 4. Later in his life, he advanced to stage 5, which is paradoxical-consolidative faith. He sought religious legitimacy in a quest for truth and justice and integrated his own identity into a particular religious tradition that inspired him to transcend himself by groping toward a more universal vision. Macolm X's overall faith then takes precedence over his moral development as advocated by Kohlberg. Faith is broader than morality, adding meaning and motivation to the moral quest for justice.

SIMILARITIES BETWEEN KOHLBERG AND FOWLER

Both Kohlberg and Fowler believe that justice or fairness in human rights is an ultimate value. From Kohlberg's definition of morality, note that he considers justice to be the central moral value. Justice is the one virtue that embodies all other virtues. Fowler considers that the ultimate meaning of justice is in the symbol of God, and that God is the center of value. Thus to Fowler the ultimate meaning of justice is equated with the action of God, which includes His symbolic reconciliation of human rights in justice.

Both Fowler and Kohlberg insist that justice must be learned within a community, a "just community" that respects human rights and treats persons fairly and democratically. Both are concerned about the quality of community in institutions such as churches (for Fowler) and prisons and public schools (for Kohlberg). The quality of life in institutions needs to embody justice and respect for human dignity and rights because all institutions teach morality or immorality, justice or injustice. Kohlberg (1967) is convinced that the school is the most promising institution for moral education, since he found "remarkably little use of religion in American children's responses to moral dilemmas, regardless of denomination" (p. 179). He is not as concerned about religious institutions as he is about moral education for justice in public schools. But Fowler is intensely concerned about both.

Furthermore, both scholars agree that intelligence or development in logic is necessary although not sufficient for development in faith and morality. An advancement in faith stages and moral stages is not possible apart from the development of the higher mental processes. Kohlberg relied on Jean Piaget's findings that intellectual growth is necessary for moral growth. Fowler, likewise, built on Piaget's stages of cognitive development, with abstract reasoning being necessary for mature faith.

Both Fowler's faith stages and Kohlberg's moral stages widen a person's social environment so that he or she becomes more inclusive and tolerant of diverse classes and traditions other than those of his or her own group. Higher stage theories are not bound by social class or ethnic differences. For example, Fowler and Kohlberg claim some of the same persons as exemplars of stage 6, such as Martin Luther King Jr., Mother Teresa, Gandhi, Buddha, and Jesus. Fowler also claims Dietrich Bonhoeffer, Dag Hammarskjöld, and Thomas Merton to be representative of a significant integration of faith and justice (Parks, 1990).

DIFFERENCES BETWEEN KOHLBERG AND FOWLER

As has been mentioned, Kohlberg believed that moral development was either independent of faith or preceded the development of faith. In an article titled "Education, Moral Development and Faith" he wrote: "Development to a given moral stage precedes development to the parallel faith stage" (Kohlberg, 1974, p. 14). Kohlberg accepted the emphasis in Immanuel Kant's thought that the religious must be accountable to the moral and to reason. Reason, not religion, provides the basis for morality. By contrast, Fowler (1976) has insisted that morality cannot be divorced from faith because faith is the motivation for "the exercise of moral logic" (p. 209). Fowler supports his position by noting that subjects may be at a higher faith stage (5 and 6) than the parallel moral stage, but the reverse does not hold true.

Another difference between Kohlberg and Fowler is that Kohlberg does not distinguish between faith and religion whereas Fowler does. Kohlberg's definition of religion at stage 3 is fairly clear because he equates the meaning of religion with affiliation in a church group. His definition at the higher stages is less clear, where he links "religious support" with religious reasoning, which supports "faith in justice" (Kohlberg, 1981, p. 318). Fowler (1989) defines religion as a cumulative tradition such as Christianity and the other six world religions. Conjunctive faith, stage 5, is created from one's own tradition and that of others. Thus faith is a broader notion than religion, and indeed at stage 6 faith is universal.

A third difference is that Kohlberg accepts liberalism as the dominant ideology of the West, whereas Fowler accepts Christian theology as basic. These divergent commitments lead to different meanings and assumptions in methodology and different content for morality, faith, and justice. Kohlberg does not argue for the universal content of liberal ideology but rather for the form of reasoning in various ideologies and cultures. Fowler, by contrast, seems to be arguing toward the form and content of a universal faith.

John Snarey (1991) has produced research that supports the notion of a universal faith and the construct validity of Fowler's faith development. Indeed, Snarey's findings "lend tentative support to the power and generality of Fowler's model and indicate that the degree of construct validity is adequate for research purposes" (p. 303).

CONCLUSION

In spite of the differences, Kohlberg and Fowler hold basic assumptions in more agreement than disagreement. Their common concern for justice, reason, logic, community, the Constitution, education, and human rights bond them together in research for human development.

Fowler's concept of faith gives breadth to Kohlberg's theory of morality. Faith is based not only on reason and rationality but on the dimensions of passion, valuing, and commitment. Kohlberg focused on moral judgment using role-taking and hypothetical dilemmas to increase moral perspective. Fowler's later interpretation of faith is linked to real-life problems and takes action as well as thought as part of what it means to be a mature adult. Although Kohlberg recognized moral behavior to be important, he did not include it in his basic theory.

Fowler, however, is vulnerable to criticism for posting too broad a definition of faith. His meaning of faith seems to entail all the functions of the ego and is so inclusive as to diffuse the distinctiveness of an understanding of faith accepted by historic Christianity. Fowler's faith is more personalistic than dependent on a particular religious tradition. Such a faith is applauded by some but criticized by others.

Questions for further research come to mind: How do Fowler's "faith" and Kohlberg's "justice" function and relate to personality development? Is Fowler's view of faith acceptable within the Christian meaning of the term? How do philosophical notions of justice correspond to psychological and religious concepts of justice and faith? Can Kohlberg and Fowler be combined as a foundation for a common morality? This last question has been addressed in this chapter. Further analysis and research would give additional input into forming a definitive answer, which should be pursued.

Chapter 3

Is the Faith of Faith Development Christian Faith?

The major research with a theological and developmental psychological perspective on the meaning and development of faith has been produced by James Fowler of Emory University and the Candler School of Theology. In this chapter, I present challenges by important critics who pose a significant question. Is the faith of faith development research Christian faith? To provide an initial answer, I offer brief summaries of some of Fowler's writings that he has listed as most important for responding to the question. I also present evidence from his writings and from the writings of other authors that he is indeed interpreting Christian faith.

A common view of faith is that faith is something one has. If I ask about your faith, you might tell me about the beliefs you hold or have. Christians repeat creeds containing beliefs. This is the content of faith. Fowler is more concerned about the form of faith in action. The emphasis is not on what one has but rather on doing and thinking and imagining. Fowler is elucidating the dynamics of faith. Obviously, psychological dynamics are functioning in faith. Hopefully, logical dynamics are operative in faith as a way of knowing. Kohlberg also insisted that logic was necessary but not sufficient for advancing moral knowing. But Kohlberg's use of the logic of certainty was too narrow for faith knowing. Thus, Fowler expanded the meaning of logic by turning it into a metaphor, the logic of conviction.The logic of conviction includes logic of certainty and extends toward a comprehensive knowing by faith. For instance, in and through faith the self knows itself, the neighbor, and God within a total and ultimate environment. In Fowler's (1986) own words, faith is:

- The process of consecutive-knowing
- Underlying a person's composition and maintenance of a comprehensive frame (or frames) of meaning
- Generated from the person's attachments or commitments to centers of supraordinate value which have power to unify his or her experiences of the world
- Thereby endowing the relationships, contexts, and patterns of everyday life, past and future, with significance. (pp. 25-26)

The self through faith knows, reasons, unites, and integrates knowledge. Here, faith functions along with imagination. Thus, faith at its highest level includes advancement in moral undersanding motivated by Christian biblical faith as evident above in the heavy reliance on biblical language such as the Kingdom of God, God's sovereignty, and covenant.

Of course, the order of these well-known stages provides the meaning and definition of faith development from the beginning of life at stage 1 to the peak of maturity in faith at stage 6. Since faith grows and changes, there is faith development. Fowler views such change as mainly gradual but accepts the more sudden and drastic change of conversions. His view is both Catholic and Protestant, especially Methodist, which includes the very dramatic conversion of John Wesley. Thus the meaning of faith evolves through faith stages, and education is the most potent factor promoting this advancement and growth of the person in faith and learning.

In summary, Fowler's (1990) definition of faith is marked by its complex dimensions. Its foundation is the experience

> of trust and loyalty underlying self and relationships. In this sense faith is a human universal, a generic quality of human beings . . . a wholistic way of knowing and valuing, . . . the unifying and life-directing response of persons . . . to the gift of divine grace. This radical understanding of "justification by grace through faith" is central . . . and . . . obedient assent to revealed truth [is central also] . . . [I]n those branches of Christianity where doctrinal formulations are understood to conserve and express directly the contents of divine revelation, faith is understood to be obedient assent to the explicitly revealed content of God's will. (pp. 394-396)

From these definitions, we can see a specific definition of Christian faith within the more general definition of faith and within the context of faith development. These introductory definitions are expanded further through the body of this chapter.

QUESTION

This chapter consists of a question and a response. The question: Does James Fowler's construct of faith meet the necessary and sufficient requirements to be Christian faith? Even after decades of research, the main question is still about the nature of faith in Fowler's work. After Fowler (1986) had read the most comprehensive evaluation of his research, he responded, "Virtually all of the essays in this collection address to some degree the appropriateness and adequacy of my use of the focal term 'faith' " (p. 280).

Major scholars on their own and in relation to professional groups have posed the question. More specifically, Bonidell Clouse notes that Fowler uses the word "faithing" and this term is not biblical (personal communication, July 10, 1990).

In addition, similar questions were posed for the prestigious American Academy of Religion. John McDargh (1984) says, "the most basic challenge that faces faith development theory in its second decade, is the critical working out of the relationship between its normative theological vision and what its psychological investigations disclose" (p. 342). Concern for the normative will lead to concern for the meaning of Christian faith.

Another important critic is Robert Wuthnow (1982), who quotes Wilfred Cantwell Smith's view of faith as distinctly Judeo-Christian compared to Fowler's view of faith. Also, Wuthnow questions whether Fowler's concept of faith is consistent with Martin Luther's. In fact, Wuthnow notes that there are no references in Fowler's (1981) index to the Bible, Abraham, Jesus, or Luther.

The *Journal of Psychology and Theology* includes more articles on Lawrence Kohlberg and Christian faith than on James Fowler. Yet Kohlberg claimed no expertise in religious studies. In fact, when religious questions were posed, Kohlberg pointed toward Fowler for a response. At least one article in this journal (Oosterhuis, 1989) does question whether the faith of faith development is biblical. For instance,

Fowler describes stages, and Oosterhuis charges that the hierarchical notion of stages is contrary to the biblical view of community.

The Religious Education Press published *Handbook of Faith*. In this book, the influential scholar H. Malony (1990) charges that Fowler seems to "reduce faith to the human search for cognitive meaning" (p. 82). Malony (1990, p. 86) also charges that Fowler advocates "functional religion" more than Christian faith. Nevertheless, Malony (1990) states that "Fowler has provided psychology with the most comprehensive model available for understanding the development of faith" (p. 89).

Religious Education Press also published *Faith Development and Fowler,* the major evaluation of Fowler's work. In it, J. Fernhout (1986) complains that there is no distinction between Fowler's faith development and general human development. Thus, according to Fernhout, Fowler does not provide a distinctive and particular definition of faith as Christian faith.

I can summarize this criticism. Fowler does not give a clear definition of biblical Christian faith, nor a normative theological vision consistent with his psychological findings. With these numerous criticisms, Fowler is vulnerable to being charged with advocating a contemporary gnosticism, that faith is more dependent on knowing than on its Object. And Fernhout (1986) charges that Fowler is not clear about the meaning of "ultimate." Thus Fowler's view of faith is vulnerable to the criticism leveled against Paul Tillich, namely, that he advocates such a broad and vague definition of faith that it includes everyone yet means nothing special to anyone.

RESPONSE

Fowler (1986a) has responded directly to the criticism by Fernhout (1986). When Fernhout reinterprets Fowler's use of the cube or cone metaphor, charging that it has no (Christian) core, Fowler offers another metaphor, namely, that faith is a precious gem which adds many facets to the meaning of faith (see Figure 3.1). Thus Fowler's insistence on the mystery of faith and his emphasis on metaphors of faith such as a gem and precious jewel are counterarguments to those such as Fernhout who charge that Fowler's approach reduces the meaning of faith. Indeed, Fowler (1991) states "that all constructive theology employs metaphor to represent the divine human relatedness" (p. 56).

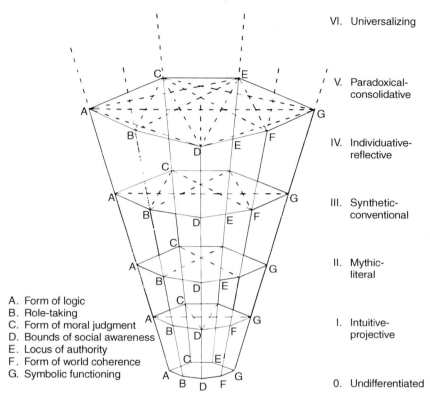

VI. Universalizing

V. Paradoxical-consolidative

IV. Individuative-reflective

III. Synthetic-conventional

II. Mythic-literal

I. Intuitive-projective

0. Undifferentiated

A. Form of logic
B. Role-taking
C. Form of moral judgment
D. Bounds of social awareness
E. Locus of authority
F. Form of world coherence
G. Symbolic functioning

FIGURE 3.1. (A-G represent structural aspects of faith in each state.*)

*The lines connecting the aspects of each stage are merely suggestive and are not to be taken as representations of empirically established relations. (*Source:* Fowler, 1986b, p. 32)

For a clear perspective, I continue to focus on just one question about the nature of faith, namely, is the faith of Fowler's faith development Christian faith? An initial answer is that his view of faith development at least includes Christian faith. Then one might wonder if Christian faith can be identified within faith development. The answer is yes. Thus our task now is to identify Christian faith within faith development research and theory. This task requires both understanding seeking faith and faith seeking understanding. Both lead to mystery and to knowledge of Christian faith. Thus some of the criticism originates from, and remains with, the complexity of Christian faith. Nevertheless, we will strive toward clarity of Christian faith in spite of the perplexing human expressions of faith. Fowler (1981) is aware of the criticism of whether his focal term "faith" meets the requirements for being Christian faith:

> these . . . are the Christian critics, particularly those who are heirs of Protestant neo-orthodoxy's stringent commitment to the Reformation's stress on faith as solely the gift of God's grace, given uniquely in Jesus Christ. . . . They claim that faith is an indigenously Christian Category. (p. 91)

Fowler's (1991) doctoral student H. Streib-Weickum (1989) reminds him of the criticism by the "Christian thinkers" (p. 118), but both assert that Fowler (1984, 1987) meets the criticism, especially in his interpretation of vocation.

Fowler (1978) identifies himself as a "Christian theist" (p. 23). He presents in his definition of faith the substance of Christian humanism as represented by Erasmus. The other half of this substance of faith is represented by the action of God in history and in the vocation of the Christian. Here, God takes the initiative in Christ and calls persons to respond by their actions in their vocation.

To be fair with Fowler in responding further to the sensitive question above, I think it is appropriate to draw the response mainly from his own writings. Thus for the source of my continued response I am grateful to Karen DeNicola, the coordinator of the Center for Research in Faith and Moral Development, and to James Fowler. His response is expressed in his particular writings that answer the question. From these writings I will summarize Fowler's interpretation of Christian faith. Karen DeNicola (personal communication, letter, July 24, 1990) listed the writings:

> one of the best references for your question is *Becoming Adult, Becoming Christian.* Jim tells me you should also review the latter part of *Stages of Faith,* Craig Dykstra's chapter in the book he and Sharon Parks edited *(Faith Development and Fowler),* and Jim Fowler's entry of faith and belief in *Dictionary of Pastoral Care.*

Although Fowler's writings are frequently enriched by quotes from the Bible, he does not lay out his theology by presenting an exposition from the Bible. In the June 1988 listing of his writings I see no specific writing by Fowler on the Bible. Whether his view of faith is biblical depends on whether we require an expository letter of the law or a meaningful letter of the Spirit. I opt for the latter along with Fowler. Fowler (1991, pp. 13, 56) is against the biblicist position, which is taking the words of the Bible literally. In fact, such reasoning is probably representative of stage 2 in his scheme of six stages. Fowler insists, as mentioned earlier, that theology, including Christian biblical theology, requires the use of metaphor. Indeed, the Bible itself is loaded with metaphors. Thus Fowler follows the Bible by constructing theology from biblical images and metaphors such as a covenant, and from biblical persons such as Paul, especially in Fowler's books (1984, 1987, 1991).

In one of Fowler's (1984) major books about Christian faith, *Becoming Adult, Becoming Christian,* he reflects on his past and present experience in midlife. Here are the elements of an autobiography and Christian faith. He is trying to discern what God wants him to do. He writes that destiny and vocation "connect our images of ourselves and of God. . . . he [Fowler] found himself mining the richness of biblical faith for images and orientation characterizing partnership with God" (Fowler, 1984, p. ix). In this representative example, the Bible is a normative source for Fowler's understanding of himself and of the Christian faith.

In contrast to the stage 2 reasoning about the Bible mentioned earlier, Fowler (1991) offers a stage 5 example of receiving a message from the Bible that broke through his deception and confusion. Fowler (1991) confesses: "The Spiritual Exercises of Saint Ignatius have been for me the most important single source of learning how to resubmit to the reality mediated by Christian symbols and story" (p. 111). He describes further how he was taught by a contemporary Jesuit how to discipline his life by entering into dialogue with the Bible through prayer.

In addition, Fowler has accepted David Tracy's (1975, 1981, 1987) interpretation of the Christian classic as an important source of texts and literature. The Bible is included within the term classic, and this provides normative sources for spelling out the meaning of Christian faith. Fowler (1984) defines a classic as "an expression of the human

spirit that seems to gather into a fitting unity something that is fundamental, recurring, and universal in our experience" (p. 79). A classic
is like the Bible and the Bible is like a classic, which includes normative literature defining Christian faith in history. Thus Fowler blends
together this meaning of classic with the Bible to form the Christian
classic and the Christian master story. Meaning is carried from classic to Bible (and from Bible to classic) and to Christian faith by way
of metaphor and analogy. To see that Fowler's faith development includes Christian faith requires that we follow his assumption and argument for his perpetual use of metaphor and image.

Additional biblical images similar in meaning to partnership include covenant, kingdom of God, co-authorship of our life stories,
and the metaphor of God as liberator. These biblical images suggest
the meaning of that faith which is integral to becoming Christian.

They also introduce Fowler's (1984) interpretation of Christian
faith in summary form that outlines the major movements of the narrative structure of the Christian classic by describing seven large
chapters in his own words:

1. *God.* "In the beginning was the Word *(Logos),* and the Word
   was with God, and Word was God . . ." (John 1:1). In the telling
   of the Christian core story, we cannot get behind this starting
   point. The principle of Being is Being itself. . . .
2. *Creation.* In the dynamic expression of Being, God gives being.
   Ex nihilo, out of and from nothing, from and by the Word, Being
   makes room for co-being. Being further differentiates itself,
   cleaves its unity, and sets free seeds of freedom and creativity
   potentiated with its own image. Generative loci of Logos are
   dispersed; the inner life of God makes room for expanded participation and partnership.
3. *Fall.* Finite freedom and vulnerability as well as the seeds of
   Freedom, grow into the illusion (and the burden) of Self-
   groundedness. Separated loci of Logos undertake to be primally
   creative, rather than participative. This results in breach, alien-
   ation, and enmity, between God and God's creation and between created beings. The image of God in the creature under-
   goes distortion and separation. . . .
4. *Liberation and Covenant.* The triune God makes initiatives of
   reconciliation. God offers liberation (from bondage, from self-

groundedness) and extends the call and imperative to reconciled partnership. God gives the gift of Way (Torah, Halakah, Law) that leads to righteousness. Then the Narrative shows us a series of oscillations between covenant and falling away, covenant and falling away, covenant and falling away, with God consistently and redemptively manifesting *steadfast love and faithfulness. . . .*

5. *Incarnation*. Logos becomes human, takes on flesh. . . . God shows forth the costly determination to restore *unity* between Creator and creature, and *com*munity between alienated and separated creatures. The intended . . . character of God's promised universal commonwealth of love is instantiated in the tangibility of words, deeds, a broken and torn body, and a remarkable resurrection from the dead. The *cross* shows in double disclosure the depth of the divine love, on one hand, and the power of evil in the defensive structures and resistance of human enmity toward God's future, on the other.

6. *Church*. Resurrection and the outpouring of Spirit from the resurrected Christ confirm and empower the Church in its calling to partnership with the redemptive and reconciling work of God in Christ and in its extension of the Christ's announcement of the in-breaking commonwealth of love. The Church is meant to proclaim and demonstrate the universal calling of humankind to covenant partnership in God's work in the world, in anticipation of the fulfillment of God's intended redemption of the world in just and righteous unity.

7. *Commonwealth of Love*. This is traditionally known as the "Kingdom of God" (Fowler, 1984, pp. 82-84).

Fowler's theology of the Kingdom and of the Church must be updated with his strong affirmation of the recent emphasis on the public church. Fowler (1987) asserts "the public church is deeply and particularly Christian. Neither Marty nor Palmer advocates some sort of religion in general" (p. 24), but all are invited into this public movement.

Some of the breadth of Fowler's inclusiveness of religious traditions is captured in the following very interesting statement. "It is in and through Christ, that we recognize the truth in other revelatory traditions" (Fowler, 1988, p. 12). As believers affirm a particular Christian faith in Christ, they also illuminate a reality of God even in other religious traditions. This faith is embodied and understood within a particular Christian tradition which reveals and conceals revelation from God. But Fowler (1984) states, "God's self-disclosure never exhausts God's being, and our apprehensions and expressions of disclosure events are never adequate fully to appropriate what is offered" (p. 80).

Although Fowler uses many abstract categories such as Being, he mainly interprets the Christian story in narrative form, which was present even in his earliest writing, such as his dissertation. Fowler's interpretation of Christian faith seems to be more theocentric than Christocentric. For example, he begins the Christian story with God and creation and then presents the incarnation of Christ. These themes are from a particular Christian tradition of biblical language and are directed toward a universal love, justice, and faith. As Fowler (1984) emphasized, "It is the character of Biblical language about the divine to use multiple metaphors for the divine-human relation" (p. 85). Stringent orthodox Christians would prefer the focus of faith to be on the deity of Christ rather than on divinity because deity is more characteristic of the biblical language.

Fowler (1986) affirms, "I have begun to see in fresh ways the deep structure of an angular, inconvenient, but tough and resiliently integral truth at the heart of orthodox Christian faith" (p. 296). This Christian faith is also expressed by Karl Barth, Søren Kierkegaard, and C. S. Lewis. Fowler (1983) asks, "what . . . are the distinctive characteristics of Christian faith? . . . Communities of Christian faith need to rediscover lively images of the theological virtues of faith, hope, and love" (p. 160). Fowler (1987, p. 24) insists that the Christian lives in community as a part of the public church committed to Jesus Christ. Fowler (1990) asserts that Christian faith is assent to revealed truth of doctrine, which is Scripture inspired. Orthodox faith is formed as the Christian community hears the Scripture, receives the sacraments, and strives to be faithful in the love of God given to the neighbor. For example, in Fowler's (1984) book about Christian faith, *Becoming Adult, Becoming Christian,* he presents a developmental, existential, and process model in which he suggests the dynamic meaning of faith in becoming Christian. Fowler (1981, p. 302; 1986, p. 283) has consistently claimed that faith development describes only the human and not the divine side of faith. His early writings are more psychological than the later writings, and the later writings are more theological and biblical than the early ones.

Fowler (1986, pp. 284, 285, 296) insists on the structuring power of the contents of faith, including the content of Christian practical theology such as its stories, beliefs, symbols, and practices. The structure and content of faith are interrelated, and each affects the other. I criticized Lawrence Kohlberg much earlier for problems in separating form or structure from content (Hanford, 1982). Fowler emphasizes the importance of the content of faith, especially in his later writings (such as those written since 1984), when Fowler's Christian practical theology is articulated. This position is supported by an excellent dissertation (Streib-Weickum, 1989, pp. 58-83). The Christian faith of faith development is expressed in the content of faith development. At least, Christian faith can be identified more in the content than in the form or structure of faith development.

Since the controversy between Fowler and his critics might illustrate the larger controversy in American society between liberals and evangelicals, I offer this chapter as a search for common ground between Fowler and evangelicals. The critics Clouse, Fernhout, and Malony are representative of evangelical concerns. In addition, Richard R. Osmer (1990) notes that "Fowler's work has received some of its severest criticisms from representatives of the Reformed tradition" (p. 51). But Osmer (1990) also shows that Fowler shares more in common than not with the Reformed tradition, such as their acceptance of the Reformed thought of H. Richard Niebuhr. William Avery (1990) also argues convincingly that Fowler agrees more than he disagrees with the Lutheran tradition. Since evangelicals accept the substance of these traditions, I propose that Fowler and evangelicals will find that they hold more of Christian tradition in agreement than in disagreement.

I offer my synoptic perspective (Hanford, 1975) for evaluating Fowler's contribution. He gives us rigorous, scientific, empirical research with an adequate guard against the main weakness of empiricism, its tendency toward reducing the meaning of the subject matter of faith. The guard to protect the richness and complexity of the subject matter of faith is provided by phenomenology, specifically the phenomenological hermeneutic of Paul Ricoeur, as suggested and developed by Heinz Streib-Weickum (1989).

Fowler's and Kohlberg's faith and moral reasoning stages can also be used to show the development from early to mature life of the quality of professional relationships. Since healing takes place within relationships and ethics is most important in relationships, we need a schema to show the distinctions required for discerning the quality of practitioner relationships. For illustration, stage 1 includes moral and faith reasoning that is normal for infants, who require ego development especially for themselves, but this reasoning might be almost pathological for an adult. The second stage is instrumental in the sense of using clients for the good mainly of professionals. They might use this reasoning when they say: We need a lot of patients going through our clinic because we must pay our bills and make huge profits.

The relationship becomes conventional at stage 3. Here, roles that entail duties increase the quality of relationships, and the practitioners are entitled to appropriate authority to act from their roles. Appeals to the law characterize stage 4. Recognizing the threat of malpractice, the physician might explain to the patient: I can only do what is legal. Please do not expect any more than the legal. Consequently, stage 5 reasoning wrestles with this problem: When is the legal moral and when is it not, and when does my faith perspective follow or transcend the law?

These tough questions must be negotiated with the patient and others to create a moral or just contract (and not just a legal contract). The contract needs to be decided with rational, moral principles of fairness and equality and with faith commitments of caring, compassion, and striving strenuously toward the good for the patient. The faith perspective is crucial for stage 6 quality of relationship because it entails movement in reasoning from contract to covenant. "Covenant" is a powerful guiding spirit taken from the biblical stories of God entering a loving (agape) relationship with persons and communities. "Conscience" as used by Kohlberg (1984, p. 44) to define stage 6 means that we know (science) with (con) moral, objective, and rational principles and we commit to the guidance of religious faith perspectives.

The late James Rest (1999) and his researchers at the University of Minnesota have shown a significant relationship between the moral and faith reasoning just discussed with the moral action or practice of professionals. Here is a frontier research challenge for integrating moral and faith reasoning with good practice. The legacies from Rest (1999) will continue to show a way of advancing this reasoning along with good practice, which is the much-needed payoff.

I have shown that in Fowler's writings his interpretation of faith is Christian. This conclusion is tempered with the full realization yet conviction of the complexity and mystery of faith. Therefore the meaning of faith is dependent upon interpretation within a dynamic process model in which the meaning of faith is changing throughout the development of personality. In this sense, faith development theory includes Christian faith. There is substantial evidence for the validity of the construct of faith (Snarey, 1991). My argument has been that the substance of the Christian faith is embedded within this construct of faith. Thus we have hypotheses for further research.

In addition, if we have confirmed that Fowler's understanding of faith in faith development is indeed Christian faith, then we can ask another hard question for bioethics: When is Christian faith therapeutic and when is it not? That inquiry takes us to Chapter 4.

Chapter 4

A Therapeutic Christian Bioethics

The meaning of therapeutic ought not be equated with popular therapeutic culture. A therapeutic Christian bioethics or medical ethics requires serious examination of two important questions. When is Christianity therapeutic and when is medical ethics therapeutic? Ruth Macklin (1993) and many others document the gap between ethical ideals or rights of patients and the reality of actual practice. This gap means that medical ethics has not yet been applied with sufficient rigor to meet the imperative to be truly therapeutic to the patient. This gap is also documented by some physicians themselves in *JAMA* (The SUPPORT Principal Investigators, 1995). Since we need a medical ethic that is therapeutic, I rely on a recognized authority, Edmund Pellegrino. In history, according to Pellegrino (1985), medicine was therapeutic when caring and curing were combined. Since his approach integrates a caring ethic and scientific cure, he has probably offered the most therapeutic approach to biomedical ethics. Since medical ethics can be derived from Christian tradition, we need to know when Christianity is therapeutic and when it is not. Christianity is effective as a source of meaning, including insight into the meaning of illness, evil, suffering, and death. Specifically, Christian faith offers hope in spite of despair, and courage in the face of death, tragedy, cancer, and other illnesses.

For two and a half thousand years, the reality of therapeutic healing has been within a relationship with a healer such as a clergyperson, psychotherapist, or a physician. Today these professionals offer caring and curing. The relationship is therapeutic when it is loving. Christian therapy is also marked by charity or agape. This broad definition of therapeutic healing includes (1) the effective treatment of illness, and (2) the careful comforting of patients in their experience of illness. Both needs require treatment by the therapeutic relationship. For example, comforting patients in their experience of illness is a major task of pastors. In addition, therapeutic treatment will include a sense of the meaning of this experience of illness and a sense of control regained by the patient. The ultimate evaluation of therapeutic healing will be decided by the good outcome of the patient's treatment. With this beginning view of therapeutic healing before us, we can ask next, When is ethics therapeutic and when is it not? Or, is ethics therapeutic when it produces a good outcome?

To achieve a therapeutic outcome, ethics must be functioning within the treatment process. For example, a purpose of medical ethics is to assist and guide a practitioner, therapist, pastor, and others toward being and acting therapeutically. For instance, an elderly man gets the bad news that he has Lou Gehrig's disease. He retires to the country and vows that he will live out his remaining days without modern technological medicine. While driving, he and his wife have a serious accident. They are rushed to emergency treatment. He finds himself within the bondage of medical technology. His wife tries in vain to communicate their story to the physician in charge. He works diligently to repair the man's body. In desperation, the couple call in an attorney and take legal action to cease treatment. Since there was not communication, consent, or contract, there was not ethical practice and therefore there was no realistic treatment or therapy. This case demonstrates the necessity of ethics for effective therapy (Carle tape, *The Right to Die,* 1985). This case also demonstrates that a particular quality of professional relationship is necessary but not sufficient for healing therapeutically.

Although almost everyone will verbally advocate the moral decision for the patient's good, we have an extremely difficult task of translating this good intention into practice because there are many goods within our pluralist society. Even though medical ethics supplies fairly clear directives about who should decide this good, power struggles and role confusion will hamper the implementation of the directives into practice. Thus the gap between the ethical rights of patients and the reality of actual practice was also documented by physicians in *JAMA* (The SUPPORT Principal Investigators, 1995). These physicians showed their seriousness about ethics by producing a massive study with over 9,000 patient subjects who were studied during a five-year period, 1989 to 1995. Serious moral problems were discovered early (1989-1991); for example, half of these terminal patients died in severe pain which could have been controlled, physicians failed to communicate most of the time, and consent procedures were not followed. The researchers were stunned by the results of this most rigorous scientific study of behavior.

The second phase of the study designed interventions to improve communication. Again, the findings demonstrated a lack of compliance in practice with the generally accepted moral guidelines for physicians. The institutional, ideological, and medical cultural forces were so powerful that improvement of moral behavior did not happen. The evidence was overwhelming that a more therapeutic medical ethic was definitely needed, according to the directors of the research, who were also physicians. These findings were so disturbing that the funding agency consulted The Hastings Center (November, 1995) to explain or at least try to understand the empirical discoveries.

Since we therefore need a medical ethic that is therapeutic, we need to know when medical ethics is therapeutic and when it is not. I am arguing that the clinical outcome should be a part of the test of the therapeutic. The other part is care. Both have been embodied and interpreted by a Christian physician, Edmund Pellegrino (1985). In history, according to Pellegrino, medicine was therapeutic when caring and curing were combined. Today, such a caring ethic is therapeutic in practice if at the same time there is effective treatment. In fact, an ethic without cure (science) could be harmful.

Pellegrino (Pellegrino and Thomasma, 1993) has offered one of the most therapeutic approaches to biomedical ethics, again because he integrates the caring and curing functions. These functions were combined for nineteen of the last twenty centuries of medicine, but during those nineteen, physicians did not have an adequate knowledge of the curing function. That knowledge was produced by the scientific method during the twentieth century but was and still is separated from the caring function. Thus Pellegrino has written several books and many articles integrating caring and curing into a medical ethics or philosophical-theological theory of medicine, which promises in a realistic way to be therapeutic.

The knowledge of caring includes compassion derived from religious traditions; especially Jewish, Christian, Islamic, Buddhist, Confucian, Hindu, and others. Caring is an active verb similar to active concern, love, and agape within Christian tradition. Caring must produce trust and needs to include curing; that is, scientific knowledge, technical competence, and skill in the appropriate or right treatment for the good of the patient. From responsible caring and scientific curing effective, treatment and practice can be rendered.

The above two paragraphs demonstrate another major contribution by Pellegrino: his integration of the two powerful professional institutions of our culture, science (medicine) and religion, personal and prophetic. Specifically, for example, he advocates that health care be available and accessible to the poor and needy.

In addition, the virtues of fidelity, compassion, wisdom, justice, fortitude, temperance, integrity, and self-effacement are also necessary but not sufficient for an ethic that is therapeutic. But the greatest virtue is love because charity is the form of the virtues, the way of life for the virtuous person and especially the professional person.

The biblical metaphor of "hospitality to the stranger" means to be therapeutic to the stranger and alien. How can we be hospitable and how can we act in a hospitable way? We might have to overcome fear and anxiety in being hospitable, for example, to a stranger with AIDS. Education can help. The biblical meaning of charity or agape and covenant can influence relationships to become therapeutic. The ultimate meaning of doing the good is that it is an act of grace such as in the Sermon on the Mount and in the Beatitudes.

Western medicine has been secular for only a few centuries, a comparatively short time when we recall the total history of Western medicine of at least 2,500 years. Since medical ethics is derived from religious and specifically Christian tradition, we need to know when religion is therapeutic and when it is not. Many theologians claim that religion, if believed in strongly enough, can solve almost all human struggles. But the problem of evil and suffering has threatened even the most devout believer. So, are there limits to the effectiveness of religion? If so, how do we intelligently draw the line to know when religion is therapeutic or not?

But a patient might not be suffering from a lack of religion but with postpartum depression, an imbalance of the chemistry in the brain. In such an experience, even with the full affirmation of faith, the patient might not be helped by religion alone. If we are not aware of these limits, we might create problems such as disillusionment about our faith and religious tradition. In addition, we might also confront the limits even of modern technological medicine. Thus, we need to understand when religion and medicine are therapeutic and when they are not. This decision requires rational, faithful, and public deliberation, which can then be embodied within a public faith. A Christian therapeutic perspective can be embodied in and through a public faith.

Chapter 5

A Public Faith

This chapter describes the exclusion of public expressions of religion from the history of bioethics during recent decades. It notes the need and the promise to include public religion for the purpose of gaining donations of vital organs for transplantation (see Chapter 6), more appreciation for the gift of aging (see Chapter 10), and more concern for universal access to health care (see Chapter 7). I also include theological support for such a program.

RELIGION, VALUES AND PUBLIC LIFE, AND BIOMEDICAL ETHICS

I am profoundly committed to interpreting religion and Christian tradition (from an inclusive, universal perspective) to call all persons to identify values to nurture and enrich public life for the development of a human bioethics. My own personal development demonstrates this purpose. When I was sixteen years of age, I experienced a dramatic conversion to Christian faith. From this encounter with Jesus the Christ, I decided to be different and to make a contribution to society. My personal and professional formation has equipped me with a humble and developing Christian faith and practice. Thirty years of studying and teaching biomedical ethics required additional competence. Now I intend to offer a religious and Christian interpretation of the gift of aging, of a responsible medical ethics, and specifically, universal health care, which is necessary but not sufficient for a civil America.

First, I am persuaded that seniors must battle ageism and neglect of older adults even within the Christian church. Then they must also create a Christian public meaning of good aging and serve the needs of a community dedicated to enunciating a public theology for a civil United States. Throughout my professional vocation I have been studying, writing, and observing the need for a public religion for biomedical ethics.

Biomedical ethics became very public during the 1960s. The emergence of biomedical ethics manifested a change in medical practice from being almost exclusively private within the doctor's office and hospital practice prior to the 1960s toward becoming more and more public. Often, moral matters must be made public before they are known and dealt with. They then become issues of public importance. A major problem for this chapter is this: as medical ethics became more public it simultaneously became less religious in the sense of drawing insights from identifiable religious traditions. Religion remained in the shadows of medical ethics; this chapter proposes to add some light.

A thesis for this research is that the emerging (from 1960 to the present) and significantly developed American medical ethics still needs a public expression of religion. While most Americans think religion is mainly private, many scholars of American religion are increasingly insisting that we need to build on private religion toward an emphasis on the public sphere of religion, the collective values of our society. Worship is an obvious example of a public expression of religion. In fact, "liturgy" means a public act of worship; an act or work for all the people, the public.

THE INCLUSION OF PUBLIC RELIGION IN BIOMEDICAL ETHICS IN AMERICA

While the first part of this proposal mentions the recent exclusion of religion from bioethics, this part explores the advantages of the inclusion again of public religion in bioethics. The previous section describes the secularization of bioethics, which the influential director of the Center for Clinical Ethics at the University of Chicago, Mark Siegler (1991), views as the problem for medical ethics. For a solution, he offers a perspective from a comprehensive history of the relation between medicine and religion. He divides this history into three ages. The age of the doctor ranges from 500 B.C. to 1965. The age of the patient is from 1965 to 1983. The age of the third-party payer such as health insurance, Medicare, and Medicaid, is from 1983 to the present.

The point here is that medical ethics needs the values from religion from the long view, especially from the first part of this history, which offers the three essentials for a good health system, namely "care, competence, and compassion" (Siegler, 1991, p. 1). This religious perspective must be included for the identity of the doctor as a caring and nurturing servant of the patient. Such values and relationship are necessary to rescue medicine from the control of the payer and from secularization. In addition, Siegler appeals to religion and theology for a source for the emphasis on the respect for the individual and his or her right to make medical decisions. Siegler is one of the three leaders (Siegler, Pellegrino, and Singer, Spring 1990) founding the new and important, *The Journal of Clinical Ethics* at the University of Chicago. Clinical ethics as formulated by Peter Singer, Mark Siegler, and Edmund Pellegrino includes a specific role for theology to function in the creation of theory and of hypotheses to be tested empirically (Siegler, Pellegrino, and Singer, 1990). Theoretical research employs the methods of logical reasoning and argument and is founded on theological principles along with other sources.

In conclusion, theologians (Tubbs, 1990) have a public responsibility to be prophetic, for example, speaking and acting as advocates for children, the poor, and the oppressed. The time is now ripe for a public religion to make its contribution to bioethics. This contribution must be distinctive to public religion and useful to bioethics. Nowhere is this faith perspective, which produces values to act on, more important than in dealing with organ donation, which is also the wave of the future, elaborated on in detail in the next chapter.

Chapter 6

Public Faith and Religion, Medical Ethics, and Transplants

Advances in technology generally have provided significant challenges to biomedical ethics. To deal with the challenge, an enlightened faith perspective informs the basic theological and philosophical issues such as the motivation and intention for organ donation (Chapter 6), the nature of human nature for the human genome project (Chapter 8), and an understanding of the power of technology as a competing faith stance (Chapter 9). I begin with organ donation.

This chapter continues discussion of the exclusion of public expressions of religion from bioethics during recent decades, offers a proposal to include the public church for the purpose of gaining donations of vital organs for transplantation, includes a brief discussion of theological support and practical suggestions for such a program, and shows the special and particular problems and promise for dealing with public faith and organ donation.

Walter Edinger (1990, p. 135) published an article on respecting donor choice in deciding to donate vital organs for transplants, and I will continue discussion of this concern. The thesis of this chapter is that the emerging (from 1960 to the present) American medical ethics needs a public expression of religion to facilitate the donation of vital organs for transplantation.

While Chapter 5 documents secularization and the recent exclusion of religion from bioethics, now I explore the advantages of the inclusion again of religion into bioethics. One effective response to the challenge of the forces of secularization and pluralism is the theological concept of the public church. The public church is "in the world but not of the world." This affirmation claims the distinctiveness of Christianity along with its acceptance and tolerance of American pluralism, which is filled with the varieties of religions. The public church provides structures for procuring vital organs for transplantation.

The public church is the church as generally understood but has a special consciousness of mission to the public, the common good. This church is concerned not only about itself but also about the needs of the pluralistic society. Some of the pluralism is within this church, which works cooperatively with other agents and forces for the good. These persons are in a partnership with God struggling against pain, loss, and death. This consciousness is expressed through the organizational structure of the church. Gandhi suggested some of the meaning of the public church in his well-known claim: he who separates religion from politics understands neither religion nor politics. The public church is both particular (Christian) and universal. It not only recruits members but calls the public congregation to meet the needs of the stranger and the neighbor. Since the public church is devoted to a particular tradition, it is not merely a representative of religion in general, civil religion, or even the church if it is neither hot nor cold, i.e., without conscience (Revelation 3:15). The theology of the public church is a strategy to highlight the normative dimension of the church. Much of the normative dimension is a theological consciousness that must be expressed through the organizational structures, top and bottom, of the public church. The normative dimension of both the church and religion is not only private and personal but also public and social. This theology of the public church prepares the church to take leadership in procuring organs for transplantation for the public good.

The notion of the public church has caught the imagination of many religious leaders. Martin Marty (1990) defines the notion to include the Catholic Church, the mainline Protestant denominations, and the evangelicals. These groups favor organ donation. "The policy of the U.S. Catholic Conference is that cadaveric transplants are acceptable" (Lyon, 1986, p. 53). Their reasonable condition is that the donor's death be determined through a responsible and definite process. Most Protestants also approve. These Catholic and Protestant groups could proceed by educating their individual congregations about their official positions. Such education could then be spread throughout the society. Since members of the congregations know and trust one another, the education would be sensitive to persons' needs. For instance, many persons might feel uneasy about considering organ donations because of their feelings about and their symbolic associations with the newly dead, especially in the case of a relative. People want their newly dead treated with respect, with bodily integrity kept whole, and treated not as a means but as an end. But the need of the neighbor for a vital organ is another important reality. If we refuse to give an organ, we express by our action that not giving is right. As churches succeed in educating their members, they will be expressing their agape (love) by their gifts of vital organs.

Mark Dowie (1988, p. 237) also informs us that even though orthodox Jews opposed Christian Barnard in 1967, today they consider organ donation to be a good and legal deed. Transplantation is encouraged and donation is a major expression of community solidarity.

Walter Edinger (1990, p. 135) documents the current shortage of organs: the supply is only about one-tenth of the demand. Additional studies (Prottas and Battein, 1991, p. 123) have shown that 75 percent of persons questioned are willing to donate. Thus, we need a program to translate this willingness into action in order to meet the need. The transplant community (mainly health care professionals) is more dependent on the public than is any other medical group (Dowie, 1988, p. 41).

Since 95 percent of organ donors are declared dead in intensive care, ICU nurses should be trained for organ procurement (Dowie, 1988, p. 134). The bereaved family members can usually be carefully approached as they gradually know and accept the death of their relative. Many wish not to have the topic introduced at that hour, but I think people can be prepared in advance, experts can assist us. For example, Dr. Stuart J. Youngner of Case Western Reserve University is an advisor for organ procurement (Dowie, 1988, pp. 135, 173). He is a source of knowledge for church communities and others on how to obtain vital organs. We need additional leaders to facilitate this process.

There appears to be a consensus in the medical ethics literature that organ donation should be carried out through volunteerism. Martin Marty (1990, p. 15) notes "that two-thirds of American citizens' volunteer hours are attracted through organized religion." These two statements suggest that the public church is the institution of choice to carry out the task of gaining a supply of organs that will meet the demand for them. Ronald Reagan advocated voluntarism, but altruism is not easily sold (Dowie, 1988, pp. 154, 195). The churches and synagogues can enhance motivation for action by providing education, persuasion, and the structures for donating organs. In these ways, religion can make a forceful public expression. These institutions are probably best suited to carry out the delicate task of being sensitive to grief and at the same time being responsible to the human need for organs.

Churches and synagogues can work with families, and the decision to donate or not usually needs to be a decision by a family. After the death of a person who has consented to donate, his or her proxy needs to confirm the consent by the deceased. Some dying persons are willing to leave the decision about donation to the family, but a family ought not override the wishes of the deceased (Edinger, 1990, p. 139).

Churches might improve procurement of vital organs because they are very influential in minority groups, especially in black communities. Presently, blacks contribute proportionately even fewer organs than whites. Blacks remain on the selection list of United Network for Organ Sharing, (<http://www.unosframe-default.asp>) (UNOS) longer, and their transplants are not as effective nor as successful. Consequently, Wayne Arnason (1991) has argued persuasively for "directed donation," that is, blacks could donate for blacks. This policy is not approved by the UNOS guidelines, but the need is so great in the black community that some new experimentation is needed. In this process, the UNOS point system, which assigns values to a list of factors relevant to distribution, e.g., need, will need to be analyzed and evaluated. Its heavy reliance on utilitarian social good criteria needs to be scrutinized. Many of these arguments for the role of the black church could be expanded to apply to the public church. The two can be complementary. Since religious beliefs have been used as a major reason against donation, education is needed to clarify and direct religious beliefs toward contributing to health and to the gift of life. If we agree with Edinger's argument for strong required request, such as a federal law requiring request by hospital personnel, then we know that persons will be confronted with the request for donation. Consequently, they will need to be ready to respond to the urgent request.

The programs of the public church could specifically include forums; insights into scripture; testimonies by recipients; education of clerics, lawyers, and funeral directors; work with curriculum writers; and distribution of materials.

The time is now for the public church to meet the need for vital organs. This idea is distinctive to public religion, useful and pragmatic to bioethics and to American society.

If concerns about organ donation are left to the individualistic character of American religion the need will not be met, because it is a large concern that requires a public response of education and community. To begin, we need public awareness of the need for organ donations.

The American public is still very confused and ambivalent about organ donation and cries out for leadership. Such a predicament is an opportunity for the public church to plan serious study and offer opportunities to explore leadership options beginning with immediate local situations. We can use research from universities and bring their experts into church communities, even basements. We can create dialogue, especially with minority communities and with physicians from various faith perspectives; clarify issues about the timing of death that would enable organs to be donated appropriately; debate the commercial selling of organs and marketing issues of organ transactions; and explore facilitating donations by those who are terminal, whose death can be reasonably predicted, and whose quality of life is not acceptable according to patient, family, physician, and clergy.

The culture wars occur around public faith perspectives and organ donation even within a particular congregation and throughout America. In addition, public conversations are needed between mainline and minority religious groups about how to proceed toward meeting the massive demand for vital organs. Fundamentalists and liberals need to be engaged in similar public meetings.

The impact of political decisions on organ procurement and distribution needs to be studied, analyzed, and evaluated with an eye toward progress. The American love-hate relation with medical science and technology needs to be exposed, understood, and dealt with in the interest of constructive cooperation on complicated issues of defining death, stem cell research, and donations by anencephalic infants, that is, infants born with no full brain but only the brain stem.

Many churches should be familiar with the National Bioethics Advisory Commission, which was created by President Clinton. We might scrutinize their approval of some stem cell research using embryos as a source of stem cells that would otherwise have been discarded. Is the opposition by some Catholic groups justified? Since the Internet offers excellent information on stem cell research, church groups could gather around the computer and discuss the issues.

These suggestions are just for the beginning of so much work that is needed. The supply of organs must meet the demand to stop the continuing tragedies.

As of July 1, 2001, the Gift of Life Agency: Transplantation Society of Michigan, reported a total of 2,479 patients awaiting organ transplants:

Kidney	1,726
Heart	77
Lung	112
Liver	434
Pancreas	130
Total	**2,479**

As of year-to-date, 254 patients received an organ transplant, 101 patients died waiting for a transplant.

Although my position thus far is predominantly optimistic, I have been challenged by a pessimistic view from a major expert in this field, Renee Fox (Fox and Swazey, 1992). Fox chose her title, *Spare Parts,* because it "reflects our increasingly troubled and critical reactions to the expansion organ replacement has undergone during the past decade—its magnitude, its scope, and the medical and cultural fervor by which it has been driven" (p. xv).

The book is developed in three parts. Part One presents the general history of organ transplantation, especially through the 1980s. Part Two describes in detail the specific artificial heart experiment Jarvik-7. Each of these parts constitutes about 100 pages, while Part Three consists of only 14 pages in which the authors present their personal story regarding their decision to leave this field of research.

The problems with Jarvik-7 greatly influenced Fox and Swazey's "new" position regarding transplantation. While I share their concerns about the artificial heart, I affirm a different perspective that includes the successful transplantations which are enhancing the lives of many recipients. Even though the book covers a wide range of impressive research, it "is not an exhaustive or even-handed work about every form of organ replacement" (Fox and Swazey, 1992, p. xv). Nevertheless, the book includes minute detail along with a thorough criticism of both the development of artificial organ technology and its ill-advised use in therapy. Both of these efforts led to the waste of scarce medical resources. Their realistic details show the psychological complexity of giving and receiving organs, the confusion of professional medical roles of therapist and investigator or researcher, and the elevated expectations of patients and families, which technology cannot adequately fulfill. Also, in certain instances the "spare parts" cannot easily fit into and operate within the complex human body.

Fox and Swazey focus on the issue of limits. They became convinced that the desperate effort involved with Jarvik-7 went beyond their notion of limits. Thus, they agree with Daniel Callahan (1987, 1990, 1993) in his three recent books that we must set limits. For example, they insist that we should limit our commitment to transplantation in favor of "far more basic and widespread public and individual health care needs in our society" (Fox and Swazey, 1992, p. 208). But I am not persuaded that we must be limited to this either-or choice. I would argue for both. For example, organ transplantation provides an effective treatment for some cancers, especially when the cancer is located in a particular organ. In addition, organ transplantation is more cost effective than some prevailing treatments. Health and political officials in Oregon might have decided prematurely to discontinue organ transplantation because of its great expense, because these treatments are now medically and cost effective. Such progress is slow.

Spare Parts deserves to be read carefully, and I regret that its authors have left this important field of study. Nevertheless, I maintain my optimism and my suggestions for facilitating especially the gift of human organs for appropriate transplantation. We need more constructive suggestions about knowing what is appropriate. The book provides a depth analysis and critical perspective from which we can assess the practice and prospects of organ transplantation. It does not directly offer criticism of the religious perspective that undergirded the Jarvik-7 project. A more critical perspective from Christian faith made public might have produced therapeutic results and a better view of limits in health care. This perspective might also have focused on justice and therefore better allocation of scarce resources.

The principle and virtue in justice are also needed to guide the fair distribution of health in managed care, as we will see in the next chapter.

Chapter 7

Mental Health and Managed Care

In this chapter, I continue the conversation going on today on the crisis in delivering mental health care within the realities of managed care. A guiding perspective is represented briefly in material from the writings of Edmund Pellegrino. He recommends the norm of patient-centered relationships to direct and govern managed care so cost can be controlled, but not by the sacrifice of quality of care. This emphasis must be balanced with a struggle for the greater social good and fair allocation of goods to all citizens. Definitions are offered along with a discussion of controversial issues and constructive suggestions to make possible a better future for the work of mental health in relation to managed care.

Alarming discussions of mental health and managed care, generally in medical ethics and specifically by D. Aycock (1996) and E. Worthington (1996), stimulated the desire in me to enter the debate. I have been teaching medical ethics for twenty-five years and have been concerned about mental health even longer. The discussion in the journal article referred to above (Worthington, 1996) seemed to suggest at times that managed care was an accomplished fact. My reading of the signs of the times suggests rather that managed care is a work in process. Although it appears to be here to stay, its exact form and structure of incentives are being determined by political and economic forces.

With the incentive of a Louis Harris poll (in *Health Affairs,* Luft, 1996, p. 33), which showed that consumers do not have a good understanding of the differences between fee-for-service and managed care, I offer a beginning working definition. In general terms, managed care represents a corporate takeover of medicine in which the medical groups of patients, physicians, and reimbursers of care are renamed consumer, provider, and insurer. A quick evaluation suggests that managed care is popular for cutting cost, but that consumers are not satisfied that their needs have been met and quality care achieved (Davis et al., 1995, p. 100). Thus, there is some urgency for us to enter the debate and perhaps help shape the future development of managed care, especially its impact on mental health.

The purpose of this chapter is to offer a normative perspective drawn from the faith and the work of Edmund Pellegrino, to further define managed care, to identify some current issues relevant to mental health efforts, and to suggest why these issues are urgent in the perspective of justice and care. This perspective may provide guidance for the future development of managed care delivering mental health services.

PELLEGRINO'S FAITH PERSPECTIVE

Edmund Pellegrino (1994a, b) provides a broad Christian perspective in which to examine managed care. The changing face of health care needs guidance from a Christian perspective such as Pellegrino's to provide focus on the emergence and development of managed care. This section identifies the nature of his perspective and sketches an outline of a position on managed care.

From the healing perspective, we can see that delivering health care requires a sensitivity well beyond simply producing a commodity, which is the general emphasis in managed care. The issue of fairness demands rethinking the economic system and procedures at work here, where economic structure needs especially to serve the healing relationship. The duties of the healer ought to be motivated by a professional relationship stimulated and defined by Christian vocation.

Pellegrino (1994a, b) is a strong critic of some managed care because too often its concerns threaten beneficence to the patient, and trust and charity toward poor patients in particular. For example, inappropriate use of the role of gatekeeping may result in a decision for financial profit over the greater good of the patient. Pellegrino justifies this criticism by his appeal all at once to Christian theology, the history of medicine, and the vulnerable predicament of the patient and what this all means or should mean to a medical professional. It is in these terms that the quality of the professional relationship ought to be sustained, according to Pellegrino.

A physician should advocate the most equitable and just system and work toward its implementation in a social setting that sets fair priorities for the good. To do this, society must define goods as ends in themselves that provide guidance and incentives for managed competition to become real managed care. Whether a society achieves this end can be evaluated, Pellegrino asserts, by the Christian and humane standard of how the society treats its most vulnerable, its children, poor, sick, and elderly. This is an appropriate end for the means of the economics of managed care, and we must guide the system directly to its end—the good of the patient. This guideline must be understood and followed because many health concerns go beyond or transcend market principles. Historically, more health has been achieved through cooperative efforts of sanitation, vaccination, nutrition, and the like than through the fee-for-service market system alone.

MANAGED CARE

The business system for managed care needs to be understood in its historical context. The supervening issue throughout this history is how to design an economic system for the humane delivery of health care. Most of this history for the last 100 years has been the story of the fee-for-service contract. This system created powerful incentives for progress but has come under criticism for overtreatment, such as the indiscriminate dispensing of medications, thereby escalating costs and sometimes producing harm. Managed care has already provided a means for curbing costs by controlling referrals and related methods. But managed care has also been seen as "mangled" care by its threat of undertreatment. This criticism is especially relevant to mental health because history shows that lack of treatment is tolerated more in mental illness than in physical illness (Sharfstein, 1995, p. 278). Such criticism can lead us toward creating a better system, a more just and humane one.

ISSUES AND STRATEGIES

We need a system that will control costs, but not at the expense of quality care, which must include appropriate care for persons with mental illness, especially chronic, serious illness. To achieve this goal, we must resolve some serious issues.

The most important need is to create a system that is directed to enhance the quality of professional relationship. This requires involving the expertise of mental health professionals. They represent an ultimate source or ideal for quality in relationships; they specialize in creating and developing such encounters. They must have legal, political, and economic support for reinforcing fiduciary duties and responsibilities.

Mental health professionals in turn should focus on the connection between mental and physical illness and show that good mental care can prevent physical illness, thereby reducing costs in very significant ways. These are resolutions that must not be left to physicians alone. They need the whole health or patient treatment team. Unfortunately, at times the AMA has protected physicians' interests, for example with self-referral, even at the risk of patients' interests (Rodwin, 1993).

All involved, from patient to professional, should work to repudiate the gag rule of managed care, the rule that prohibits full disclosure to patients of treatments, that withholds information necessary for informed consent by the patient. Instead, we must advocate wherever possible transparency of informed consent, that is, full disclosure, with open, frank, and candid conversation to achieve authentic consent. This advocacy will reinforce the legal action taken nationwide by states to outlaw the gag rule.

I propose that we consider the following additional strategies: recommend equality of care between medical and mental health care and assertively enter this debate within society; align with psychiatrists, for their Council on Psychiatry and Law (1995) (Hogue, 2001) affirmed fiduciary obligations to patients, patient participation, access to appropriate psychiatric care, and quality of care in health care systems; insist on economic incentives that maximize health, including mental health value; challenge insurance companies to pay for mental and other therapies, stressing the needs of children, and demand that all children be included in health insurance; remind insurers of the source of their funds, mainly from working people, as their contracts will show; scrutinize critically the interaction between health and economic values; join forces for academic excellence, which will support therapists who are competent and effective; distinguish between religion that heals and religion that does not.

Some mental health professionals might need to reevaluate their offer of free or inexpensive counseling. What does this practice communicate to a secular world where charity means "cheap" and real value is money value, where "free or inexpensive" may communicate a lack of real value? We need to know the value of care and ask if benefits have actually been rendered. If there are no benefits, then there is no real value, even though the service is cheap (Wells, 1995, p. 81). Sigmund Freud memorably insisted that patients were helped by participating in their treatment through paying for it.

Should therapists work with seniors to make sure Medicare includes their services? From its beginning, Medicare provided some funding for mental health for seniors, but Medicare remains a fee-for-service system, according to F. Miller (1996). There are Medicare health maintenance organizations (HMOs). In 1995, 5 percent of Medicare patients were enrolled in HMOs; in 1996, 10 percent, according to Lewin and Jones (1996). We need to compare Medicare with managed care enterprises and compare the 10 percent on managed care with the rest of those enrolled in Medicare. We must remember that Medicare will remain the main market for managed care well into the future (Etheredge, Jones, and Lewin, 1996, p. 96), and that important studies show that seniors are not satisfied with HMOs.

Prior to the creation of Medicare in 1965, much of the insurance industry, many employers, and the American Medical Association denied health insurance to retirees and other seniors. To correct this, Medicare was created.

Mental health professionals should explore appropriate strategies for dealing with lifestyle and lifestyle changes in health care, psychotherapy, and managed care. E. Morreim (1995) shows the increased attention to the relation of lifestyles and managed care in the present and posits as much again for the future. In this evidence, we see the promise of managed care providing a strong incentive for preventive medicine and ethical concern.

Hospital ethics committees ought to guide managed care toward ethical imperatives for creating, maintaining, and sustaining quality care. Religious mental health practitioners should help Americans deal with death, and in less expensive ways. G. Annas (1994) shows that Britain and Japan show less intensity of anxious concern about death, and as a consequence their health costs are less than half of ours. Death anxiety drives the commitment to technology, which in turn drives costs upward. Here, too, quality of care must provide guidance for economic policy.

Concerned professionals might form a nonpartisan, issue-oriented advocacy group for parity for mental health services. Specifically, they might offer suggestions to the Department of Health and Human Services and to the president. The rationale for this political activity is clear: former President Clinton proclaimed the need for a consumer Patients' Bill of Rights so that managed health care does not become poor health care. He believed that cost could be reduced and quality still maintained. On balance, this seems to be happening in some HMOs. If there is no success in legislating a Patient's Bill of Rights, Americans may need to face up to the hard question: Is the insurance mechanism the best way to deliver health care?

If these general guidelines could be firmly enunciated at the federal level, then appropriate priorities and policies might be implemented at the state and local levels. In September 1996, Congress agreed to expand mental health coverage to people with group health insurance. But companies with fewer than fifty employees are either excluded or exempt from this requirement. Problems remain because, as R. Hungate (1996, p. 11) insists, "the cost of care, not its quality, is the dominant driver of change."

AN UPDATE ON ETHICS IN MANAGED CARE FOR THE TWENTY-FIRST CENTURY

Before describing the current context of the controversy surrounding ethics in managed care, I present a sample test question and a recommended structure for clinical case analysis in bioethics that will primarily show the importance and seriousness of this controversy. The test question is: Select a case from a standard textbook in bioethics, or from a clinical experience, or an issue and analyze the moral problem, principles, position, and other important aspects of the case. State the reasons you agree or disagree with the position in the textbook, or in other sources. What experiences helped you improve your thinking on this case?

To begin, I will briefly present a case from real life that is especially pertinent to ethical problems in managed care systems. Prior to

1987, John McGann found himself a job at H&H Music in Houston. He was probably happy with his contract, which promised AIDS-related health coverage for $1 million. But in 1987, he was diagnosed with the AIDS virus and was informed by his company that they had switched their health plan to a self-insurance plan and that his $1 million coverage was reduced to $5,000. In 1992, the Supreme Court even refused to hear this case, which then had the practical effect throughout the country of making such drastic changes in a contract not only legal but even potentially constitutional. Lawrence Kohlberg (1981, pp. 154, 227) considers an appeal mainly to the law to be typical of stage 4 reasoning. When there are conflicts such as whether the law is moral or just, then the conflict should be settled by an appeal to the American Constitution, basically a moral document, which includes postconventional principles. Kohlberg claims this reasoning to be characteristic of stage 5. The Supreme Court's justification rested on the federal Employee Income Retirement Security Act (ERISA), which originated in 1974. The title of this legislation appears ironic, if not deceiving. Such insurance is legal and cheaper for companies with 500 or fewer employees, which affects about 40 percent of all employees, according to *Newsweek* (Shenitz, 1992). More than a decade of tolerance of this legislation has elapsed, and employees with not only the AIDS virus but also with multiple sclerosis, cancer, and other such diseases have died. The law still stands with little hope of political will to change in spite of the cost in suffering and death.

You (the reader) and I can first identify not the technical but the ethical problems. There are obvious, though not typically recognized, moral problems surrounding the contract. For example, did McGann know how easily the contract could be changed so significantly? Can a contract judged legal even by the Supreme Court be immoral? What happened to McGann's rights and autonomy, and where was the compassion for the critically ill? Where was the connection between love and justice? Here, we refer to moral, reasonable, and objective philosophical and religious principles, which is the second step following identity of moral problems in an ethical case analysis.

The third step is to take a position that must be justified by reference to relevant ethical principles. My discussion of the Supreme Court represents one position. They decided basically that the employer's decision was right because it was legal. On the other hand, an editorial in *USA Today* (Walker, 1992, p. 12A) declared that "Congress must close the loophole which allows employers to cut health benefits for sick employees." Also in 1992, President William Clinton would have agreed with the editorial when he proposed health insurance for all workers. This second position is still being debated. Which position is more right or less wrong according to moral principles derived from philosophy and religious traditions?

If we follow logically the above three steps under rigorous guidance and practice, evidence especially from the late James Rest (1999) and others shows that we can advance our moral reasoning even on such difficult cases and issues as this one.

Within the current context, we can continue to practice on the following positions on ERISA. First, the American Medical Association argues for ERISA reform to make health maintenance organizations, a subset of managed care organizations (MCOs), accountable and even legally liable when the HMOs make medical decisions. The point is to make managed care accountable just as physicians are made accountable by liability for malpractice. Such a position is extremely important, because an inordinately large number of errors in the health care system have recently been reported in the media. The AMA joins with patients who cry out that they are not protected against errors until patients can sue HMOs. In addition, the AMA is troubled that the gag rule (which prohibits practitioners from discussing more expensive treatments even when they are medically indicated) is still required by some HMOs. Moreover, the AMA, through their spokesman Don Polmisano (an MD and attorney who appreared on C-SPAN, January 14, 2000), insists that market forces cannot correct malpractice. Thus, the AMA in 2001 favors the Senate's Patients' Bill of Rights and asserts that the patient can ration care. And here in Michigan, Governor John Engler favors a Patients' Bill of Rights (C-SPAN, January 19, 2000). But which one?

President Clinton wanted a Patients' Bill of Rights passed in the year 2000 because the lack of health insurance is the seventh greatest cause of death in America, and 82 percent of the uninsured are workers. Thus, according to C-SPAN (January 19, 2000), health care as an election issue ranked second among voters, especially their three concerns about (1) the uninsured, (2) Medicare, and (3) HMOs and patient rights. Americans want incremental change, moving away from only employer systems (in which the employer is the main source of health insurance) toward individual rights, specifically the rights of patients.

The following three authorities, appearing on C-SPAN (January 20, 2000), favored more health insurance coverage. President Clinton continued incremental change by specifically requesting additional coverage to include long-term care. Another Democrat, Ron Pollach, a major player in this struggle, sought common ground for support for CHIP (Children's Health Insurance Program), that is, more coverage for children which began in 1997, passage of Patients' Bill of Rights, and more support for Medicaid which assists 4 million Americans. Chip Kahn, an advisor to Republicans, famous for his TV commercial featuring Harry and Louise, and head of Health Insurance Association of America (HIAA), favored Clinton's incremental proposals. Thus, Kahn led his private insurance associations in cooperation with Clinton's public efforts.

A position that contrasts with all three above was espoused by Tom Donohue, the national president of the Chamber of Commerce, on C-SPAN (January 14, 2000). He approved managed care, as it is, which he said is indeed the greatest health care system in the world. He recommended expansion of ERISA to further protect small businesses. He would increase market forces, lessen malpractice claims because they increase costs, and make government liable. He cautioned Congress against legislating to allow any more suing of HMOs.

In summary, this controversy continues into and beyond 2001. The Republicans promise solutions from the private sector, the insurance industry. The Democrats promise solutions from the public sector such as in the expansion of Medicare and incremental moves toward coverage for the 13 million children without coverage. All age groups in the American population are crying out for greater access to affordable health care. Our hope is in the faith perspective, as enunciated by Pellegrino, which will provide the motivation for the political will to respond to the crying need.

CONCLUSION

Since expert evaluations of managed care range from considering it the *problem* in health care to considering it the *solution* to the problems in health care, mental health professionals need to offer their own distinctive evaluation, showing the advantages of parity for mental health with physical health and contributing their perspective for managed care to produce quality care for the future. I call for a faith perspective to deal also with genetics in Chapter 8.

Chapter 8

Ethics in Genetics:
The Human Genome Project

Since the Human Genome Project is the most ambitious research in genetics, it has the potential to shape life in the twenty-first century. This new technology is already creating new ethical and religious issues. I discuss three of these issues. First, did the Congress of the United States make a good decision by committing us to this project for the past fifteen years? Second, will this research and technology change the basic nature of human nature? Third, will this knowledge be used to discriminate against persons? Constructive analysis and recommendations are offered to deal with these important problems and opportunities.

In the *Journal of Interdisciplinary Studies,* Robert Blank (1989) presented an article titled "Human Genetic Intervention: Portent of a Brave New World?" Since research in genetics doubles every two years, much has happened since 1989. The most important occurrence has been that the U.S. Congress allocated 3 billion dollars over fifteen years toward the mapping and sequencing of genes in the Human Genome Project (HGP). Actual funding appropriation commitments are only made year by year. Three percent of the funds are allocated to study the ethical and legal implications of the project. This is the most money ever allocated for biomedical ethics.

First, should such a large investment in the HGP have been made? Bernard D. Davis (1990), along with his department at the Harvard Medical School, has provided a main challenge to the "big science" status of the HGP. Davis was not convinced that the project would produce enough benefit to justify its funding "at a level equivalent to 20 percent of all other biomedical research" (p. 342). However, this argument about the size of the appropriation can also be developed in comparison to projects outside biology. Thus, the entire HGP costs less than the Hubble telescope. The savings and loan debacle was projected at 500 billion dollars. Three space shuttle engines are 2 billion dollars. Certainly this controversy affects not only scientists but also society as a whole. The issue is about priorities in the allocation of scarce resources. The project has produced knowledge about how to diagnose, treat, and even prevent diseases. But this knowledge might lead and direct research toward additional high technology medicine, and there may be more pressing needs now.

Such needs may be found not only in genetics but also in the health environment. Thus, we need a program to meet such health environmental problems as babies being born underweight and cigarette advertising, which contributes to the increase of lung cancer. Troy Duster (1990) persuasively describes this concern.

Second, the HGP may affect, perhaps adversely, our understanding of human nature. Thus, before his resignation, the Nobel Prize winner and chief executive of the HGP, James Dewey Watson (1990), claimed that the project might reveal the essence of human nature. This claim poses profound psychological, philosophical, and theological questions about the nature of personhood and troubling questions about what portions of the scientific community understand the essence of human nature to be. Was Watson assuming that the essence of human nature will be dependent on genetics? Is his assumption reductionist? That is, does he reduce the worth and dignity of personhood? Does he assume that a person has no intrinsic value that transcends his or her genome? Is our worth and dignity not more dependent on being created in the image of God than on genetics? If we assume that human nature has theological and moral dimensions, then we might not want to risk losing those dimensions by taking chances on genetic experimentation and engineering under the control of those who might share Watson's implied reductionistic understandings of human nature and personhood.

Third, the HGP still poses potential threats of morally unjustified discrimination between persons. For example, geneticists working on the HGP produced tests for diagnosing diseases. In fact, these tests provide the initial practical impact of the research on society. One troublesome impact will follow from the fact that some persons in society discriminate against those diagnosed with genetically based diseases. This tendency toward prejudice is exacerbated by confusion about the meanings of genetically based disease and health. Since there is a long-term gap between the development of the technology for diagnosis and the subsequent development of appropriate treatment, there is a danger that many people will be stigmatized by the use of diagnostic tests and will not benefit from any treatment.

Americans need to be prepared to prevent these abuses by adhering to a prima facie (almost absolute, self-evident) obligation to hold all genetic information in strict confidence. This obligation must be met unless it conflicts with other equal obligations. Health insurance companies and employers have to lessen or eliminate their demand for diagnosis so that this confidence can be honored. Unfortunately, there is not an international consensus to protect confidentiality of diagnoses. This serious problem demands attention in the near future.

Conversations with genetic counselors indicate that there is also a need to be reminded that the patient has a right not to be informed. Some counselors feel a legal obligation to disclose all information. But some genetic information, such as disputed parentage or Huntington's disease, could be devastating to a client. Thus, the parties will need to discuss and come to an agreement about whether all information must be disclosed. Thomas Caskey (1991) of Baylor College of Medicine in Houston suggests that presymptomatic test results not be made available to insurance companies and employers.

The work on the HGP must be made available to the public. John C. Fletcher (1991) advocates that public discussion be directed toward a national consensus on issues. In addition, he recommends that these deliberations be continued to gain international consensus. Such consensus is very elusive due to problems such as the following: Americans and others do not know whether commercial corporations will allow their genetic research results to become public. Many persons in India approve sex selection in reproduction, but most Americans disapprove. Discussion of genetics in Germany is intensely controversial due to the painful memories of Nazi abuses of genetic research. Dorothy Wertz and John Fletcher (1989) have produced extensive research to help us move toward greater understanding and perhaps an international code of ethics for guidance. Peter Singer (1991), editor of the journal *Bioethics,* has applauded this massive research data from 682 geneticists in nineteen countries.

Religious groups have provided leadership toward dealing with the ethics in the Human Genome Project. A major source of this leadership has been J. Robert Nelson, the former director of The Institute of Religion in Houston, Texas. Nelson, Hessel Bouma, Thomas Caskey, and others created two conferences of leaders in medicine, philosophy, and religion from 1990 to 1992. Over this three-year period, they studied genetics, religion, and ethics. From the first conference they produced four substantial papers and a book (Nelson, 1994). Their insights have been disseminated to the mainline Protestant denominations, Orthodox Christians, the Catholic Church, Jewish doctors, Islamic scholars and physicians, a Hindu scientist (attended the conference), and other leaders in religion and science (Nelson, 1994). This work provides a model for becoming informed about the HGP, identifying ethical issues, and taking steps toward benefiting from the promise of the HGP. At the first conference in Houston (March 30-April 1, 1990), John C. Fletcher offered the following five guidelines:

1. Disclose all clinically relevant information to patients, family, and appropriate significant persons.
2. Confidentiality is very important but not an absolute guideline.
3. Options for parents (even including abortion) should be safeguarded and held in strict confidence by medical geneticists.
4. No sex selection.
5. Genetics service programs should be voluntary. Since not all medical insurance provides prenatal diagnosis, this service, plus counseling, peer support, and information in newsletters are provided by voluntary organizations and are listed in the Directory of National Genetic Voluntary Organizations.

These guidelines and others can provide substance for our conversation toward an ethics in genetics with special relevance to the Human Genome Project.

In 2000, the Genome Project completed a draft of the human genome. Let us ponder for the future one of its findings that all people have 99.99 percent of the same genetic structure.

On Monday, June 26, 2000, President Clinton announced the completion of the working draft as a wondrous achievement. The director of the HGP, Dr. Francis Collins, added that knowledge had now been disclosed that had previously been known only to God, hinting at Collins' faith perspective. But in inevitable American style, half the stage was taken by a representative of private industry asserting boldly their success. The proud representative was Dr. J. Craig Venter, president of Celera Genomics (their Web site is <http://celera.com>). This intense competition between public government and private corporations documents ongoing controversy between these powerful political centers. The private corporations demand patents for their present discoveries and even for anticipated findings into the future. These aggressive actions are counter to policies of the American Medical Association, who banned patents by physicians in the early twentieth century (see Chapter 9 for details of this heroic story).

The progress of the HGP marks not only a continuation of controversy but also new beginnings for a revolution in medicine, and perhaps its transformation. Medicine already has greater expertise in the all-important task of diagnosis because of the HGP. Diagnosis will lead to treatment advances in cancer, heart ailments, and hundreds of additional disorders and maladies. New medications or drugs are coming forth. In fact, Venter is promising individualized prescriptions. He plans to correct the practice of general prescriptions for all persons in broad disease categories. His research is intended to prescribe specifically and only to those patients who will be helped by an individualized prescription.

The HGP has additional important implications for biomedical ethics in the twenty-first century. Suppose a woman becomes pregnant unexpectedly after age thirty-five. Some experts would predict that her baby would have a 20 percent greater probability for some major genetic disorder. Such a prospect might persuade her to abort. Prenatal therapies might give her very precise predictions and even treatment of the fetus, which might convince her to carry the pregnancy to term. But, we must not be overly optimistic, because gene therapy has not lived up to its hyped promise. Such confusion shows the need for genetic counseling. Should it proceed as value-neutral and thereby nondirective counseling? Gwen Anderson (1999), a leading genetic nurse at Stanford University, has produced effective qualitative socio-psychological research challenging the assumption that the counselor should be nondirective. In addition, a cofounder of the Hastings Center, Willard Gaylin (2000, pp. 31-33) and a psychiatrist, Glenn McGee (1997, p. 93), agree that value-neutral psychotherapy or genetic counseling are not possible or certainly not probable. McGee leads the pragmatic approach to bioethics, which is compatible with my interpretation of a faith perspective.

Chapters 6 through 8, on managed care, organ donation, and the HGP, need to be understood within the history of religion, medicine, and technology. Chapters 10 through 12, focusing on the elderly, pastoral care, and nursing, also require knowledge of the historical development of medicine, especially of medical technology, in Chapter 9. Moreover, we will see that technology is an issue in itself.

Chapter 9

Faith and Medical Technology: Toward an Ethics for Medical Technology

In this chapter I sketch an overview of the history of medical technology from 1880 to the present. From this historical development, research questions and sources of information about those questions are presented. The later section of the chapter focuses not only on the technologies but also on ethics for medical technologies. The conclusion includes questions from this review for further research.

INTRODUCTION

Definitions

An inclusive definition of medical technology is appropriate for this survey of research questions and literature. Audrey Davis (1981) considers medical technology "to signify the physician's use of instruments, devices, and appliances in the diagnosis and treatment of disease" (p. 3). Davis (1981, p. 245) elaborates this definition further by discussing one of the most important books on medical technology: *Medicine and the Reign of Technology* by S. Reiser (1978). A third major historian of medical technology, Joel Howell (1988), defines medical technology as simply the machines that physicians use.

Lewis Thomas (1974) defined high technology as "the genuinely decisive technology of modern medicine exemplified best by methods of immunization against . . . various virus diseases, and the contemporary use of antibiotics and chemotherapy" (p. 99). High technology is the result of basic scientific research, which reveals the mechanism of disease. This science is different from a narrow applied science. In addition, high tech is different from low tech, such as artificial insemination, which has been practiced for centuries.

NINETEENTH CENTURY

Physicians struggled through the nineteenth century with little success in treating patients until near the end of the century. The mainstream MDs began to have phenomenal success in treatment at the beginning of the twentieth century, which continues to develop in the twenty-first century. Physicians often moved from general practice to specialties, and even created new technologies and new specialities. For example, the ophthalmoscope was used especially in developing the first (in 1917) new specialty—ophthalmology. About one in four physicians was a specialist during the early period (1880-1930) but four in five physicians were specialists between 1930 and 1980, according to Reiser (1978).

In reflecting on the need for these early technologies, Howell (1988, p. xvii) and Davis (1981, p. 11) emphasized the importance of technology for being precise in diagnosis, for example, using a thermometer to measure the process of fever in the body. Davis (1981) stated:

> Measurement of physiologic and anatomic characteristics, especially body temperature, volume of air inhaled and exhaled, the pressure of the blood in the arteries, the rate of the beat of the pulse, sensitivity to pressure and pain on the skin, sensitivity to colors, sounds, and tastes, and the tension in the eyeball were among aspects of the human body described with the aid of numbers. (p. 11)

This historical development was not smooth and easy. For example, the ophthalmoscope was the focus of contention between general practitioners, ophthalmologists, and optometrists. At first, ophthalmologists claimed the ophthalmoscope as identified with their special competence. But some optometrists and even opticians could use the ophthalmoscope. They frequently reminded physicians that many general practitioners were not competent in the use of the ophthalmoscope. In addition, by 1913 George Crampton developed the battery-handled ophthalmoscope, which made it a practical instrument for internists, neurosurgeons, and many other practitioners. Ophthalmologists tried to claim authority to interpret observations made using the ophthalmoscope, but this claim was not firmly established. Eventually, ophthalmologists established themselves as a specialty within the AMA and specified that ophthalmologists would practice medicine including treatment of eye disease and injuries to the eye. The definition of the practice of optometry did not include the treatment of eye disease and injuries to the eye. Optometrists could refer patients to ophthalmologists for their treatment. Even the authority to refer was an achievement for optometrists, thus the establishment of ophthalmology as a specialty when the AMA solidified their exclusive authority.

J. Bronzino and colleagues (1990, p. 11) assert that the most significant innovation for clinical medicine was the X ray. This technology enabled the physician to see bones and thereby diagnose fractures and experiment with treatment. In addition, the lungs could be viewed. Since X rays must mainly be done in the hospital, this technology changed the location of treatment from the home to the hospital, and the hospital was becoming an institution of actual treatment around the turn of the twentieth century.

The following is a specific example of the struggle of physicians during the early period. Doctor George Dock (in Howell, 1988, p. 282) tells us the importance of X ray technology. "The dream was, and still is, to endeavor to detect and treat the disease, instead of treating the patient." Such a statement would be severely criticized today, when treating the disease is often taken for granted. But Dock is writing in 1921, when he was thinking of his experience of trying to treat a patient when he did not have X rays to identify pneumonia. In Dock's time, a general practitioner might try to treat the patient without X rays. He is also telling us about the importance of specializing in medicine, or at least working with X ray technicians who could implement the technology to treat the disease and thereby really help the patient. Also, Dock emphasized that the technician assists him. Finally, Dock describes his role in teaching medical students to use X rays and diagnose disease.

As a second example, hypertension requires a technology for its diagnosis because it produces almost no symptoms for the patient to report to the physician. Shortly after the introduction of the technology to measure blood pressure, insurance entrepreneurs quickly

learned that the device could measure longevity due to the relationship of high blood pressure to mortality. This early experience is similar to current concerns about the difficulty in predicting the many
uses of valuable medical technology.

Here is a third example. Railroad employers quickly obtained the
ophthalmologist's technology and used it to identify and thereby
screen out applicants who were color-blind. Thus the pattern emerged
early that medical technologies were used for many purposes their
creators or inventors never imagined. Simultaneously, these technologies and specialties contributed to the success of scientifically trained
physicians throughout the twentieth century.

TWENTIETH CENTURY

If you contacted a physician in the nineteenth century, you would
have little assurance, if any, that you would get better. This predicament changed significantly in the twentieth century. Many historians
such as Davis and Howell give credit to the innovation of medical
technologies and specialties for achieving effectiveness in medical diagnosis, prognosis, and treatment.

No Patents for Physicians

Davis (1981) writes

> Although physicians developed a special technology, they did
> not adopt all of the customs and practices associated with other
> technologies. One practice physicians condemned was applying
> for a patent on an instrument invented by a doctor. The medical
> profession almost unanimously frowned on physicians and sur-
> geons who sought patents for instruments and devices they had
> invented. The American Code of Medical Ethics included a pro-
> vision against owning a medical patent. . . . Dentists frequently
> obtained patents . . . a practice that helped to maintain the . . .
> gulf between the medical profession and dentistry. (pp. 240-241)

Such an unusual commitment of fidelity to a profession provided a
solid foundation for the power of the American Medical Association

to be exercised throughout the twentieth century culminating in this profession becoming supreme among professions.

The Power of the American Medical Association

The AMA was founded in 1846. In 1904, the AMA formed a permanent Council on Medical Education, which established standards for scientific education and thereby grounded the authority of the profession. Indeed, the AMA promoted not only science but also the social class of physicians in their emergence as a sovereign profession.

The AMA demanded strong commitment to professional development at the turn of the twentieth century and became a powerful organization. It provided professional journals, most obviously the *Journal of the American Medical Association,* for the publication of advancements in the new medical technologies. New therapies were presented, reviewed, and evaluated. The AMA also became the political advocate for the profession. It established standards and requirements for the new specialties, which were typically accompanied by new technologies. Since the specialists usually created the new technologies, both tended to be identified with professional competence. If this connection holds true, current policy makers should keep this historical development in mind as they debate the trend toward mainly training primary care physicians, sometimes at the exclusion of training specialists, because history seems to show that they are a major source of innovation and competence.

Technology Replaces the Personal Relationship Between Patient and Physician

The leading authority on medical technology in America is probably Stanley Reiser. Davis acknowledged Reiser's leadership at the beginning of this chapter and praised his contributions to the history of medical technology. He also holds leadership by editing an international journal of technology assessment. Reiser (Reiser and Anbar, 1984) asserts an important criticism of technology:

> Increasingly, practitioners encounter patients for relatively brief and intermittent periods—such as the consultant visiting a hospitalized patient whom he or she has never before met. In such

visits the technical aspects often dominate, for there is no time or prior relationship to determine much about who the patient is, or what the patient thinks about the illness or the needs it engenders. And even in medical relationships that are not so discontinuous, technological measurements and measures tend to crowd out other dimensions of evaluation and therapeutics. . . . That which is unique in a patient's illness can often be learned best by non-technological inquiries based mainly on dialogue. . . . To the extent that inordinate fixation on the technical aspects of medicine diminishes the possibilities for or the importance of person-to-person dialogue, we become less effective in meeting illness. The triadic relationship of practitioners, patients, and machines is one of the most difficult of all associations to master in health care. (p. 17)

Biomedical Ethics Stimulated by Technology

Most writers in biomedical ethics insist that the threat of technology initiated biomedical ethics. Many books and articles begin with concern about new technologies and new medical research. Some others attribute the perplexity not as much to the technology per se as to the influence of the technology on the roles of practitioners. Reiser's discussion provides evidence for this view. Still others point to the pluralism of American culture, which always creates confusion for moralists attempting to communicate to very diverse audiences. Thus there is need to understand medical ethics within its historical context and its relation to technology. Within this historical development, we need to understand the nexus between medicine and science, science and technology, technology and medicine, science and religion, medicine and alternative medicines, and science and values or ethics.

USE OF THE TECHNICAL-ETHICAL DISTINCTION

The first step in thinking analytically about biomedical ethics requires that we clarify the technical-ethical distinction. Although many bioethicists use this distinction in setting up problems, I doubt that physicians and others trained with a heavy emphasis on science and technology readily make the distinction. For example, I know that Jack Kevorkian does not make the distinction and appears assured that he has created a good technical solution with his "death machine" to provide a comfortable process of dying. This technical solution solves the moral problem to Kevorkian's satisfaction. Joanne Finkelstein (1990, p. 13) expressed the point more generally: "Indeed, so highly valued is technical knowledge that it can supersede moral considerations and argument in providing a base upon which therapeutic and research decisions are taken."

Troubling Abuses of Medical Technology

In his book *The Troubled Dream of Life,* Daniel Callahan describes technology replacing nature in the control of death. Callahan's (1993) specific complaint is that

> [t]he process of dying is deformed when it is subject to the violence of technological attenuation, unduly extended by medical interventions, directly or indirectly.
> Technological brinkmanship is the most common way of creating the deformity—that is, pushing aggressive treatment as far as it can go in the hope that it can be stopped at just the right moment if it turns out to be futile. That brinkmanship, and the gamble it represents, can both save life and ruin dying; this is the dilemma it poses. The most obvious kind of technological violence comes when a particular course of treatment—some forms of chemotherapy for cancer, say, or cardiopulmonary resuscitation (CPR) for a dying person—itself directly imposes the violence. (p. 192)

Some suggestions toward the ethical use of technology are:

1. Ask the hospital ethics committee to evaluate the prospects and consequences of the use of a new technology.
2. Screen technologies through the process in which new medications are studied, evaluated, and decided.
3. Study the motivation for which a technology is offered and give priority to the motivation of benefiting the patient over profit making.

Relevant to these suggestions is the fact that former President George Bush signed the Safe Medical Devices Act on November 28, 1990, which expanded the authority of the Federal Drug Administration to regulate medical devices.

Vincent di Norcia (1994) offers a useful method for ethical analysis of the use of technology. Since most technology is now produced by large organizations, he recommends that the stakeholders evaluate as soon as possible the negative impacts of a technology in relation to its Social, Economic, Environmental interests and human Rights (SEER). SEER provides a standard of values as the bar of judgment of a technology. Since serious problems often occur when organizations have already invested heavily in the production of a technology, he provides a description of the six stages typically involved in the production of a new technology. The stages are innovative breakthrough, development and variation, wide diffusion, mass use, maturity, and decline. If evaluation is rigorous in the early stages, changes can be made before heavy investment. This method had advantages over the usual late utilitarian calculation, which would determine the useful value and social consquences of the technology only after huge investments had already been made.

Religion and Technology

Is technology a religion in American culture? The use of technology in health care sometimes blocks healing and at other times facilitates healing. Our challenge is to use the biblical tradition to discern when technology is healing or not. Ian Barbour's (1993) *Ethics in an Age of Technology* provides enough of the meaning of the biblical religion and of technology to clarify when the use of technology and tradition is healing and when it is not. Barbour (1993, p. 8) presents moral and religious values relevant for an appraisal of technology.

Although Barbour (1993, p. xviii) concludes that technology has been adequately dealt with in medical ethics, I question whether medical ethics has adequately dealt with technology and biblical religion since medical ethics has not generally dealt very much with biblical religion. In spite of or regardless of Barbour's conclusion, his book presents valuable material, especially background material and information on the natural environment, which are significant for biomedical ethics. Even more specifically, he relates biblical Judeo-Christian religion to technology. For example, Barbour (1993) notes the appropriate balance between technology and power (pp. 15, 18,

21), idolatry and religion (pp. 41-61, 146), technology and the future (p. 179), and technology assessment and the future (pp. 223, 261).

Barbour's work is extremely helpful in presenting the contribution from religion to technology. He offers insights from competent academic research in philosophy, religion and theology, and science. He is a trained physicist. Although he interprets the distinctive and authentic theological values from the Jewish and Christian (East and West) sources, he also includes meaningful guidance for technology from other religions. While his perspective is broad, his theology is particular and sophisticated, namely a biblical process theology. For these reasons, his thought on technology was the focus of further academic work at the Annual Meeting of The American Academy of Religion in Chicago, November 1994.

Technology Assessment

We need to present, analyze, and evaluate technology assessment. We also need to understand the role of values in relation to the use of technology and its assessment within health care. Ought all technologies be tested by random clinical trials? The Congressional Office of Technology Assessment found that only an estimated 10 to 20 percent of the techniques that doctors use are empirically proven to be effective (Office of Technology Assessment, 1978, p. 7). This provocative judgement is confirmed and explained by the wisdom and seasoned judgement of Arnold Relman, the retired longtime editor of *The New England Journal of Medicine,* now a professor at the Harvard Medical School. He explains that much of medical practice and technology is untested or inadequately tested because new technologies are introduced so rapidly that the evaluation process cannot keep up. The needed testing is certainly difficult and would be unethical from the perspective of protecting human subjects. Thus even skilled clinicians frequently do not have adequate information to know which technologies are worthwhile. Many controversial technologies and theories of medical treatment are beyond the reach of the Food and Drug Administration. Relman (1979) offers constructive suggestions. One is that major health insurers budget more funds for more thorough evaluation of new technologies. This investment would enhance both the interests of the insurance companies and the public. In addition, Relman is convinced that we have too many specialty physicians. Their practice tends to escalate costs of technology and limit the personal relationship between practitioner and patient. Relman notes that the latter need requires attention, especially by physicians. He even recommends that physicians be paid by salary so they would be freer to enter and cultivate meaningful and therapeutic relationships.

Finally, Relman offers his definition of technology, which is consistent with the definition adopted by the U.S. Congress. His definition is, "Any discrete and identifiable device, substance, procedure, or facility, used for the diagnosis, treatment, or prevention of disease" (Relman, 1979, p. 1444).

Clinton's Futile Opposition to Physician Specialization

The Clinton (1993) health reform plan did not deal with technology and did not give attention to the use of technology in American health care. The book *The President's Health Security Plan* does not even include a reference to technology. Is technology the driving force increasing the cost of health care? Many experts answer yes and argue that increased use and cost of technology is due to the increased number of specialty physicians. That is, specialists tend to create and use increasing amounts of technology.

The Clinton health care reform sought a significant reduction of specialization among physicians. Instead of the present percentage of specialists (80 percent), the reform called for 50 percent. I will explore this issue from the history of the medical profession, which can be analyzed according to three points:

1. Specialization is firmly embedded in the history of medical professional development from 1880 to 1980.
2. Competence in medical practice is linked to specialization and to competence in the use of a particular technology. This specialty competence was an improvement over the competence of the general practitioner.
3. The professional identity of the physician is defined by his or her specialty. Indeed, specialties were created from innovations in technology. Ophthalmology emerged from the invention of the ophthalmoscope. Radiology emerged from the discovery and use of X rays in medicine. Technology contributed to the amazing success of medicine that was realized in the twentieth century.

Evidence shows that knowledge needed by the physician for diagnosis and treatment has been derived from technologies used by specialists.

CONCLUSION

In conclusion I proffer questions for further research:

1. What are the reasons why some technologies fail?
2. What is the phenomenological reaction of patients to various selected medical technologies?
3. What does Daniel Callahan mean by "nature," which is replaced by medical technology in controlling death?
4. What is replaced in question 3—technology or the ideology behind the technology or the ideology about death?
5. What does Christian faith say about the meaning and therapeutic practice of dealing with "natural" or tragic death in health care?
6. What is the impact of technology on the treatment of the elderly (see Chapter 10)?

Chapter 10

A Faith Perspective on the Elderly in Bioethics

Our pastor asks regularly at the beginning of worship: Are there announcements of celebrations? The most common responses are the announcements of birthdays, but adults usually do not disclose the age of other adults, especially not that of women. Fortunately, this experience is normally transacted with humor, but it could also exemplify subtle age discrimination. If so, we need firmer affirmations of aging. Suppose we stand up in church and say, "I turned forty yesterday. Praise the Lord for another year of growth." After all, since we are children of God, doesn't God expect us to grow up? I think so.

Since there are many more serious facts of age discrimination, even culminating in elder abuse, and our problem is in our perspective, this chapter offers a faith perspective on accepting aging and affirming the elderly. First, we need to understand the history of our negative view. Second, I present a developmental vision, psychological and theological, of the human life cycle. Third, I offer a sample course on bioethics and the elderly and consider some of the current issues for the elderly in bioethics such as setting limits on health care for the late years, exploring the complexity of futile treatments.

HISTORY

Attitudes toward the elderly have changed from positive to negative attitudes in American history. These changing attitudes are traced here from the colonial period to the present.

Colonial

The Puritans projected a positive attitude toward elders and the elderly, especially as they were perceived to be exemplars of righteousness and wisdom. For example, the seating charts for churches included a seat of honor for seniors close to the pulpit. This elders' bench honored the aged. Then too, when colonial clergymen grew old they did not retire. Moreover, inheritance was by primogeniture, and the eldest son inherited the estate or home. Colonial people would round off their age to the higher year, for example, claiming to be forty when they really were thirty-nine. Colonials named children after their grandparents in the seventeenth and eighteenth centuries. During the eighteenth century, dress emphasized age, as in the wearing of white wigs.

Modern

Certainly by the nineteenth century and industrial times, there was change in the churches. The elders' bench was rented: therefore, wealth replaced age as the badge of honor. The wig was tinted brown and the toupee was introduced. After 1880, the older worker was not viewed as efficient after age forty-five to fifty. After 1890, pensions were a way of getting rid of old workers, making room for the young. The elderly were not valued because tradition was not valued. This meant also that teaching an academic commitment to religious tradition was not cherished.

This modern period, 1850 to the present, projected a negative attitude toward old age according to the predominant view among historians and sociologists. Donald Browning's (1980) definition of modernity (pp. 109ff.) is useful for understanding the predicament of the elderly in contemporary society. Browning (1980, pp. 13-39, 109-113, 119-128), along with C. Lasch (1978), associates modernity with narcissism. A commitment to narcissism means denigration of old age, because narcissism includes an emphasis on the self only and is youth oriented. Lasch interprets narcissism to be the result of capitalist competitive individualism, which produces a marketing orientation to personality. The narcissist attitude toward sex is not Puritan but permissive. The narcissist lacks interest in the past or the future and fears death and growing old. Lasch agrees with psychoanalysts that we need the loving memories of the past and the resources of history. Narcissists try to live for themselves only in the present moment. They are separate from the continuity of the generations and of posterity, and their commitment to popular therapeutic techniques replaces religion. Thus, narcissism is devoid of moral motivation.

Browning (1980) considers narcissism only a part of modernity. Thus he interprets modernity by his descriptions of psychologies that have become cultures. Specifically, psychoanalysis relies too heavily on science for control. B.F. Skinner relies on the environment and a reinforcement schedule to control people. Carl Rogers and others in the psychology of joy believe that modern technology controls people too much. Browning continues this diagnosis into the twenty-first century and suggests a treatment from William James.

CONSTRUCTIVE THEORIES FROM WILLIAM JAMES, KOHLBERG, AND FOWLER

James

What kind of persons must or ought we be to live effectively in modern society in spite of its predominant narcissism? If society is narcissistic, moral motivation is lacking and thus is desperately needed. James' psychology of culture differs from narcissism. He advocates caring between generations. This view of the caring psychology (especially the emphasis on generativity by Erik Erikson) is an antidote to narcissism and a source for a healthy interpretation of personality for all generations. James' strenuous mood, a strong, intense feeling of being moved, driven by a moral imperative, provides the source of motivation for being moral and the faith or ethics of belief for doing the moral action. His altruism, meliorism (a belief that the world is improving), and freedom supply sources for motivation. According to James, being free means being responsible and thereby motivated to risk heroic moral action for the good. Thus James presents an alternative to narcissism, because he strikes the balance between freedom and control. He blends the ethical and the mystical to provide a prudent rhythm of life in relaxation and in strenuous efforts, which make the difference in creating the good.

James embraced an existential attitude of choice, decision, and risk, which is clearly present in his ethics. Since James is so creative, inclusive, and idiosyncratic, it is very difficult to identify his position. His ethic is a mystical altruistic rule utilitarianism and a humane religion.

James is more definitely teleological than utilitarian. His teleology is evident in his strong reliance on evolutionary theory, his pragmatism, and his openness and optimism about possibilities in the future. His strenuous mood and life includes a deontological "ring" or "bite." So, James includes both the teleological and deontological attitudes among his multiple dimensions of thought on ethics and a synthesis between the ethical and the mystical.

Henry S. Levinson (1978), in a Princeton dissertation, argues that a concern for salvation is dominant in James' thought. If so, then the mystical or salvation would override the ethical. But I think James' theology emphasizes the strenuous life, which is both moral and religious, each penetrating the other. More specifically, James affirms the ethical imperative of Puritanism but rejects its determinism and moralism, and he discusses ethics as being inclusive, compassionate, and altruistic.

James selectively appreciates Puritanism. He advocates caring for generations, a source for a healthy interpretation of old age. His attitudes toward personality and therefore the elderly counter or challenge the Calvinist Puritans yet also make a significant contribution to a moral philosophy, psychology, and theology. This interpretation of aging and the aged is consistent with his life. James was born in 1842 and died in 1910. Thus, he lived sixty-eight years, which was beyond the average life span for his time. Forty-seven was the average life expectancy around 1900. His personal and professional life provides an ideal for moral development of the elderly and the elder as moral exemplar. He was able to move through and beyond depression to integrity and wisdom, and moral purpose such as Erikson describes in his eighth stage of development. James was concerned for the optimal future in his reinterpretation of tradition and of the strenuous moral life. While Kohlberg chooses John Dewey as a moral exemplar, I add William James because he was aware of the hazards of technology and was one of our greatest public philosophers.

In summary, James' ethic included metaphysics, the phenomenological and the empirical, selections from utilitarianism and Immanuel Kant, personal identity through moral achievement, relaxation, existential choice, a sense of the tragic, democratic pluralism, a limited God, wholeness of body and mind, aesthetics, conversion, reform or protest, cognitive reason and emotion, evolution, pragmatism, anticipation of Jean Piaget and Kohlberg, socialism, religious motivation of mysticism and saintliness, and selected Puritanism and secular modernism. James created, even in his last years, when he wrote *Some Problems of Philosophy* (1911) and *A Pluralistic Universe* (1909), and we might recall that his first publication of *Principles of Psychology* (1890) has not been surpassed by anyone, in the sense of presenting a creative, depth interpretation of the meaning of human personality.

Kohlberg, Fowler, and the Life Cycle

A particular perspective on the life cycle will certainly influence, if not decide, whether aging is a positive or negative process. The modernist projects a linear theory of human development. The line gradually goes up, symbolizing our work and professional advancement to a peak age when we earn our top salary. Next, the line begins to curve downward. This point can represent downsizing, retirement, and other factors showing our decline in productivity or reflecting age discrimination. Now, we plummet downward toward unworthiness. This linear view is a powerful source of the negative view of aging and the life cycle in our society.

In contrast, Kohlberg (and Fowler) offer positive viewpoints of the life cycle. Instead of a line, Kohlberg's theory might be pictured as a cone similar to an ice cream cone. Our world horizon opens up and becomes wider as we grow. This step by step or stage by stage advancement also needs growth in responsibility from self to family to community to nation to the global community. Since Kohlberg's hard data limit him to five stages, he leans on Erik Erikson's stage 8 for generativity and integrity and Fowler's stage 6 of universal faith to hypothesize the highest stage characterizing the elderly. Fowler's (1981, p. 319) data are also limited, but he notes that his only representative of stage 6 is a senior, an eighty-year-old Catholic monk (Fowler and Keen, 1978). Although we are in soft or qualitative data, we do have a potentially positive metaphor for growing old. Thus Kohlberg (1973) in *The Gerontologist* states, "That adult moral stages might exist is suggested by the fact that moral change is clearly a focal point for adult life in a way cognitive change is not" (p. 499).

Kohlberg (1973, p. 500) views the task of achieving integrity as basically religious, religion broadly defined. Such integrity connotes not only moral integrity but also integrity of meaning and is therefore religious and philosophical. This existential meaning of integrity includes awareness of death and the problem of evil and injustice such as Job experienced in the Bible when he wrestled with the problem of suicide. Such questions require metaphysics and the use of metaphor to explore answers, as in the philosophy and mystical experience of Plato and Spinoza, according to Kohlberg. In contrast, Kohlberg (1973, p. 501) considers Erik Erikson's stage 8 to be culturally relative and not a strict structural, logical, and moral stage. Kohlberg's colleague, Robert Kegan (1982, p. 28), considers integrity of meaning at early stages of development, which is still another view of this important construct.

Kohlberg (1974) suggests that moral principles do not require faith for their justification. Their justification depends on the consistency between principles and practice or action, as among stage 6 religious persons who integrate moral principles consistently with their performance. Thus religious faith functions to motivate the integration of principles with action.

Stage 7 is Kohlberg's most controversial stage, probably because it deals with religion and has the least evidence compared to other stages. Since his research is dependent on longitudinal data, stage 1 has the most factual support and stage 7 has the least. Indeed, he is reluctant to call 7 a stage because it does not meet criteria to be defined as a stage. Thus, he opts for calling 7 a metaphor, perhaps following Fowler. Stage 7, then, is like the following characterization. Stage 7 describes the end point of human development. In this sense, it is the most important achievement producing the fulfillment or completion of our journey. Kohlberg insists that we must achieve the moral purpose of stage 6 to move into 7. In addition, there are psychological tasks and challenges such as a functioning generativity. For example, a grandparent nurtures and generates growth through a rich relationship with a grandchild. Since Kohlberg's colleague, Erik Erikson, developed eight stages, Kohlberg drew meaning, especially of integrity, from Erikson's view of the last phase of life tasks. Integrity called for the full maturity of ego strength to battle and hopefully overcome depression. I believe this struggle was personal and existential for Kohlberg. Also, Kohlberg alluded to Job in the Bible as an illustration of the suffering in late life which required religious meaning from transcendent sources. Stage 6 was understood as humanistic but 7 was cosmic and mystical. Exemplars were Spinoza and John Dewey. Specifically, Spinoza believed in moral principles, science, natural law, and the union of the mind with the universe. Many Catholics found Kohlberg's emphasis on natural law to be very appealing because it was rational and universal.

Stage 7 persons have the strength to act on universal principles by living according to them. Stage 7 persons have the strength to act on universal principles of justice even in an unjust world. Kohlberg (1973) suggests that John Dewey, who in his seventies wrote *A Common Faith* plus *Art and Experience,* might be representative of Stage 7. D. Boyd, a productive doctoral student at Harvard, was the first to suggest to Kohlberg that John Rawls, a major moral philosopher at Harvard, represented stage 6. Ernest Wallwork (1980), outstanding moral philosopher and social scientist at Syracuse University, notes that "Kohlberg believes [that] Rawls most faithfully represents stage 6 among contemporary philosophers" (p. 287).

Additional positive images are embodied in exemplars of moral development such as Albert Schweitzer, Mahatma Gandhi, and Erik Erikson. The significance of the elderly in moral development is that they represent the final stage of development as we know it and thereby represent empirically the goal of development and the personal virtues (according to Erikson) necessary for growth and moral maturity. Such exemplars are important for professional development, as suggested in the following question. What is the source and nature of the influence of elderly professionals who exert moral imperatives for other professionals and for professions? An example of such elderly professionals is Leon Jaworsk of the Watergate hearings: "I am 69, do you really think I am still building a career image?" (Gutmann, 1980, p. 445).

A SAMPLE COURSE ON BIOMEDICAL ETHICS
AND AGING

Course Description

My course on biomedical ethics includes the issue of cultural values and aging. The course has, in fact, contributed to shaping humane

cultural values of dignity, justice, compassion, autonomy, and beneficence in relation to health care. Medical ethics is a field in which one
can become fascinated with new mind-boggling technological advances. Yet the humane substance seems to be in traditional religious
and philosophical concerns of care, justice, covenant, trust, liberty,
and fidelity, especially in relationships. These values and virtues
need to be interpreted in new ways and in relation to the technological
so that the technological will serve human life.

We need not only to keep up with new knowledge in an expanding
field but to maintain clarity of perspective about the significance of
the new research. For example, most illnesses derive from societal
causes, e.g., war, poverty, malnutrition, and other such problems.
Thus the causes of illness and its treatment have their origins and expressions in ethical issues of justice, equality, dignity, and utility.

Paul Ramsey argues that Christianity has shaped medical ethics
and much of the meaning and interpretation of law and public policy.
This is true when the validity of Christian ethics is established outside
and within Christianity. Also, does Christianity provide a necessary
and sufficient approach to ethics and medical ethics? I think the answer is yes for Ramsey, Childress, Pellegrino, James Gustafson, Lisa
Cahill, Sondra Wheeler, William F. May, John Kilner, Richard
McCormick, Ian Barbour, Stephen Post, David Thomasma, Gilbert
Meilaender, and Alastair Campbell. Many others can be included in
this list, such as those in professional groups including the Society of
Christian Ethics, The Center for Bioethics and Human Dignity, American Society for Bioethics and Humanities, and The Park Ridge Center for the Study of Health, Faith, and Ethics.

Introduction to the Course

An anecdote told by Robert Butler (1975) of the National Institute
on Aging is an example of ageism in the denial of the pain of the elderly:

> There's the story of the 101 year old man who complained of
> pain in his left leg. "Morris," said his physician, "what do you
> expect at age 101?" Morris replied, "But my right leg is also 101
> and it doesn't hurt a bit. Now explain that." (p. 182)

Ageism is an issue: How do we accept our own aging? We can begin with self, deal with time, and show organic relations between generations, and especially reflect on ethics and ageism. The course focuses on ethics and the elderly.

A major purpose or function of ethics is to protect persons such as the elderly. Ethics is similar to law in setting forth principles, rules, and guidelines for maintaining fair treatment. Within medical ethics, there is much more literature on protecting fetuses, children, prisoners, and the mentally ill than there is on the protection of the elderly. The elderly are a major group in need of protection. Seniors confront many additional moral problems such as their relationships with their family, fair allocation of health resources, including prescription medicines, discernment of futile treatments, and physician-assisted death or suicide. Some practitioners avoid elderly patients because they are viewed as too slow and therefore consume too much time. Approximately 2 million older adults are abused and maltreated annually throughout America.

Course Outline: Specific Objectives for Biomedical Ethics and the Elderly in a Faith Perspective

In the course, teacher and students will accomplish the following:

1. Distinguish and describe the relation between technical and ethical aspects of a health-related issue, problem, case, and decision. See the introduction of this book.
2. Provide a framework of moral principles, theories, values, and faith viewpoints in order to construct critical positions on bioethical problems, cases, and policies. Also, we will study metaphors to complement principles.
3. Name defining characteristics of a moral professional-client relationship related to faith.
4. Discern when medical ethics and faith commitments are therapeutic and when they are not.
5. Describe a moral problem, a faith perspective, and a justified position on the problem within a health-related case and issue.

In this chapter I discuss only objective 2.

Objective 2: Principles

Identify moral principles that are relevant and pertinent to moral issues of ageism and the treatment of the aged in health care. More specifically, identify such moral principles and issues within actual cases, personal and professional. Analyze the issues by reasoning about them in relation to the moral principles. Make provisional decisions of what ought to be done and justify the decisions by appeal to facts, principles, and logic. For example, the obligation to obtain a patient's informed consent is justified or constituted by the principle of respect for persons. Moral principles are constitutive of, and give guidance for, moral obligations.

Thus, we will study these questions: What values or principles have what impact on the aged? What ought the cultural values be for a healthy interpretation of aging and of the aged? More specifically, what moral principles are most relevant for an ethics of health care for the aged? The following five moral principles are suggestive and representative.

1. We begin with respect for persons as interpreted by Lawrence Kohlberg. Is such respect dependent on age? Kohlberg considers the principle of respect for persons as primary. John Rawls considers it secondary or derivative but important, and Ernest Wallwork (1980) considers the principle as distinctive of the Judeo-Christian tradition.

Also, Alan Donagan (1977, p. 239ff.) insists that respect for persons is substantially the same as agape, as in Gene Outka's (1972) study of agape. The additional standard principles include:

2. Autonomy
3. Beneficence
4. Nonmaleficence
5. Justice

Translations of the Golden Rule or Principle Toward a Common Morality for America and the Teaching of Ethics

America needs a common morality. Presently, this concern is best dealt with in *Prospects for a Common Morality* edited by Outka and

Redder (1993). This important book offers translations and interpretations of the Golden Rule as a source for a common morality. The Golden Rule appeals to justice for all (p. 11). For example, the Golden Rule reflects Augustine's confidence that what persons want for themselves does not vary across cultures. In fact, the Golden Rule can articulate the universal essence of the moral life. Various translations of the Golden Rule appear in all of the major religions. This claim is cited by W. Spooner (1914). The Golden Rule does not tell us which actions to perform, but it does provide a way to judge actions. Augustine interprets the Golden Rule as an appeal to interpersonal consistency and a willingness to test our actions by reversing roles. Yet Augustine's convictions influence his interpretation or translation of the Golden Rule. For instance, Augustine prefers the translation in negative form, "That which to thyself thou would not have done, do not thou to another." "What thou art unwilling to suffer, be unwilling to do" (Outka and Redder, 1993, p. 117). Augustine also adds the New Testament Greek for "good" to the meaning of the Golden Rule, and he shows that the rule would prohibit lying. The rule sets limits on our interests and encourages us to promote the interests of others as we do our own. Finally, Augustine writes a rich interpretation of love and the Golden Rule.

Also, philosophers write to interpret the Golden Rule, which shows its presence and relevance to the secular world along with the religious. Alan Gewirth (1982) offers good criticism on the various translations of the Rule.

In summary, our task will include at least the following for objective 2:

1. Knowing the moral principles of respect for persons, autonomy, beneficence, nonmaleficence, justice, and others which are pertinent to health care for the elderly.
2. Applying these principles to cases such as in the example where we must clarify and decide what our moral obligation is in obtaining a patient's consent.
3. In cases where age might be used to cancel the usual rights, then the use of age cancels needed protection of the aged, who are vulnerable to hasty decisions for death—especially when they are poor.

Metaphors

While we can define ethics as reflection with moral principles, ethics is also reflection with moral metaphors. Kohlberg, Fowler, and James Childress (1997) accept metaphors and narrative as ways to see the mystery of the moral life. Metaphors require a modification of universal principles of logic such as noncontradiction. Metaphors are contradictory when taken literally, for example, "man is a wolf." The literal meaning is absurd in many such expressions. Thus the symbolic or analogical meaning transcends the usual rules and principles of logic. Such transcendence is necessary for meaning because language is fundamentally metaphorical. Thinking and reasoning drive persons to use metaphors consciously or unconsciously, and perhaps profound truth is metaphorical, including that truth ultimately produced by science and theology. Meaning requires a shift, twist, or revision of interpretation. Are metaphors and narrative a valid source for normative ethics? I think so. They might not be simply true or false, but they are vital for meaning and values. Metaphors create similarities and generate meanings. Our picture of the world is influenced by the metaphors we project to describe it or to prescribe the world we think ought to be, e.g., the Kingdom of God. Metaphors bridge old with new knowledge.

Metaphysical views require analogy and metaphor to think from the familiar to the mysterious unfamiliar and vice versa. Our capacity to think abstractly of metaphysics presupposes metaphors. Metaphors present and represent perceptions or pictures. Sigmund Freud showed that metaphors stimulate and represent perceptions or pictures along with free association and have important meanings in case work and study. Freud and Ian Ramsey knew that models and metaphors provide insight.

The metaphorical sense is looser or more transcendent than the legal sense. This realization facilitates understanding the seriousness of the ethical, because moral problems require more than a legal framework, namely a framework including principles, metaphors, and models. A model is a more general metaphor. The model used to identify illness will influence, if not determine, the model for the professional role. For example, the mechanical medical model of disease determines the professional role of the doctor as a supermechanic of the body.

The Bible is filled with rich, meaningful metaphors such as a covenant, hospitality, body of Christ, "I am the vine, you are the branches," shepherd, father, mother, Kingdom of God, and many more. These can be grasped by our imagination through faith and not only guide but also motivate moral action.

Outline of Biomedical Ethics Dealing with Ageism and Aging

In the course, present actual cases. Doing ethics of cases without principles is blind. Doing ethics with principles without cases is empty and too abstract. We need a dialogue from abstract principles to concrete cases and then from cases back to principles for justification. This list offers options for the dialogue:

1. Katz, Capron, and Glass (1972), in a massive book, *Experimentation with Human Beings,* presented a case that aroused interest in medical ethics. A physician, Richard M. Ratzan (1980), in *Hastings Center Report,* has studied the specific parts of the case that deal with ethics and the elderly. Ratzan (1980, p. 297) writes: "In 1963 two researchers and the director of the Department of Medicine at the Jewish Chronic Disease Hospital (JCDH) in Brooklyn injected patients with cells that contained cancerous material. Many of the issues raised by this case have been broadly debated—problems of informed consent (there was significant doubt that these patients had ever been told that the cells were cancerous) and beneficence (the research was in no way related to the patients' care). However, one important aspect of the case has received less attention: these patients were institutionalized and most were elderly. The general question raised by the case is: do the elderly, simply by virtue of their age, constitute an especially vulnerable group of potential research subjects that requires special protection?" (p. 32)
   Ratzan (1981, p. 297) documented that "it is naïve to think that any subject, especially an elderly one in an institution with all its subtle forces of paternalism, institutional coercion and dependence, makes a decision about participation in research, especially a non-therapeutic" research. Thus, non-therapeutic research with the elderly should probably be prohibited.

2. Sally Gadow's (1980) article from *The Gerontologist* includes three cases focusing on special problems with the elderly and on two principles, autonomy and beneficence. Two of Gadow's cases are from Robert Veatch's *Case Studies in Medical Ethics* (1977).

3. Consider a case of a seventy-three-year-old man who will die because of gangrene in his leg if he does not have the leg amputated. Since he refuses consent for the amputation, what should be done? The disturbing response from some of my students was: well, he is seventy-three. Their decision was determined by age, and they had difficulty seeing that such a decision would be blatantly unfair.

4. Additional biomedical ethical issues related to the elderly:
   a. Just allocation of health research and service. The research ought to enhance the life of the elderly. They are entitled to a fair distribution of research and service. For example, research on arthritis and senile dementia is important for the elderly.
   b. Theft of belongings from elderly persons in nursing homes and in home care services.
   c. Since the elderly might not have relatives to give proxy consent, there is a need for advocates for the elderly in health care.

One very important class session will be spent going through the article by Sally Gadow. We will follow her analysis of a case, its facts, the images of the aged, the moral principles, and the relation of these parts of a case analysis. After we have mastered the process of analysis, we will work on other cases. In addition, we will review significant literature that deals with ethical issues and the elderly. In twenty medical ethics textbooks which I have reviewed, more pages are devoted to prisoners than to the elderly; the elderly have not been given adequate attention. Here are examples of neglect of the elderly:

1. Richard M. Ratzan searched through *Index Medicus* from 1975 to 1981 and found only six articles dealing with medical ethics and human experimentation including elderly subjects.

2. I add the *Journal of Health Politics, Policy and Law,* which committed almost all of Vol. 6, No. 1, 1981 to health policies for

the elderly. For example, "reluctant" best describes health professionals' attitudes toward caring for the elderly (p. 62).

3. The most widely used text, *Principles of Biomedical Ethics,* by T. Beauchamp and J. Childress (1994), does not list "elderly" in its index.

4. *The Textbook of Health Care Ethics* by E. Loewy (1996) refers to only three pages under "elderly" in its index.

5. Other resources for dealing with the needs of the elderly:
   a. Guest speaker: Moral issues from the White House conferences on aging.
   b. Guest speakers: Congressman of the House Committee on Aging and a senator from their Committee on Aging: Moral issues relevant to the aged.
   c. Colleagues
   d. Play: *Shadowbox*—about dying in a hospice.

6. Bibliographies and books for the teacher of biomedical ethics and aging:
   a. *Journal of Health Politics, Policy and Law,* vol. 6, no. 1, 1981.
   b. Veatch, Robert (1979). *Life Span.* Veatch edited this book, which includes an eight-page bibliography of articles and books on the values relevant to interpreting the life span of human development.
   c. Van Tassel, David (1979). *Aging, Death, and the Completion of Being.* Philadelphia: University of Pennsylvania Press.
   d. *Bibliography in Bioethics* in many annual volumes from 1974 to the present.

Assignments

1. Readings:

   • Current articles from *Hastings Center Report, The Gerontologist,* and *Journal of Health Politics, Policy, and Law.*
   • Beauchamp and Childress (1994). *Principles of Biomedical Ethics.* This is the best textbook presentation of moral principles in relation to health care.
   • Howard Brody (1981). *Ethical Decisons in Medicine.* This is the best text by a physician for physicians.

- Ann Davis and Milo Aroskar (1997). *Ethical Dilemmas and Nursing.* This is probably the best text by nurses for nurses. I suggest that nurses read Brody's text and premeds read the Davis and Aroskar text.
- R.N. Butler (1975). *Why Survive?* This paperback is still a good summary of the plight and predicament of older persons in our society.
- May Sarton (1973). *As We Are Now.* A short novel that presents a sensitive impression of experience in a nursing home. Look for moral issues and relate moral principles to thinking about the issues.

2. Collect additional current cases on medical ethics and the elderly. Type them and turn them in to the professor. By "additional" I mean in addition to what is already presented in the course materials. Identify moral issues and principles in your cases.
3. Visit housing for the aged.

There are additional issues to study, such as the rights of the elderly within nursing homes. In response to complaints of abuses, the federal government in 1999 offered regulations to protect the rights of elderly residents. For example, the regulations attempted to give control of visits to the residents instead of the staff of the nursing home. The regulations also limited "transfer trauma" by making transfer voluntary and insisting that there be preparation and counseling for a transfer. Where the government contributed funds to nursing homes, it had power to enforce such regulations. Yet the regulations were only partially successful in limiting harm. Regulations alone cannot effectively implement beneficence, compassion, and respect. A meaningful faith perspective is needed for states to provide funds, inspectors, and action for stronger enforcement.

Another issue is that Medicare excludes payment for routine eye care. Since the elderly need this service more than other age groups, the nonpayment hurts them financially. This decision needs review in relation to the principle of justice or fairness.

Although children are given age-related information in taking drugs, the elderly are not. Yet the need is great among the elderly because they often have several medical problems simultaneously. Overmedication is so prevalent that Dr. Joseph Foley (1981), of the medical faculty of Case Western Reserve University, considers drug poisoning as frequently the main cause of presenting symptoms. Moreover, the information on the drugs is generally not readable by the elderly because of small print and other such problems. More research on drug interactions in the elderly is also needed. Physicians, pharmacists, and others need to be sensitive to these and other special problems of the elderly. The uncritical reliance on the *Physician's Desk Reference* needs scrutiny.

Bias against the elderly is an issue of justice. For example, while in the United States a young person would be selected and granted priority for lifesaving treatment over an older person by medical practitioners for utilitarian reasons (when not all can be selected), in Sweden and other cultures the older person would probably be selected.

Evaluation

1. At the beginning and end of the unit, describe, in writing, your impression and knowledge of the process of aging and of the aged. The specific purpose is to compare attitudes toward aging and the aged at the beginning and end of the unit.
2. Present to students a case from health practice. Ask them to identify the moral dimension of decisions, issues, and conduct in relation to the process of aging and the aged. Next, instruct students to list moral principles relevant to the case. Give an exam at the beginning and end of the unit and have the student compare and evaluate along with the teacher.
3. Evaluate the course with the use of objective, standard measures of moral reasoning, e.g., the Defining Issues Test (DIT).
4. List readings, assignments, etc., and ask students to rate which were the most or least helpful or useful for learning.
5. Do some of this evaluation at the middle of the process.
6. Consider the following questions at the beginning and ending of the course:

   - What is the effect and worth or value of a medical ethics course? Were behavioral changes stimulated and manifested?
   - What objectives can be reasonably achieved?
   - What content of curriculum should be selected?
   - What teaching strategy should be used?

- Should the teacher primarily facilitate group discussion, as suggested by Kohlberg's research?
- Should the course be team-taught to implement the interface of the academic with the clinical? Example: including a nursing professor.
- What lecturers, films, etc., should be integrated into the learning experience?
- Should visits to clinics, hospitals, etc., be included?
- Should ethics be taught as a separate course and/or integrated into the total nursing and allied health curriculum?
- What negative effects should be eliminated from the medical ethics course?

CONCLUSION

The Buddha experienced conversion when he confronted an old man close to death. This vision revealed and shaped the Buddha's own future. The Christian quest for salvation and conversion was and is decisive for me. But all of us can integrate Eastern thinking about human development as passing through a confrontation with death and despair to an "enlightenment." There are examples from faith in stage 6, from Western Quaker Christianity, and from the mystical writings in the Judeo-Christian tradition that show a passage through despair, "the dark night of the soul" of St. John of the Cross, to a sense of love for God, a love that overflows into agape and service to other human beings. This kind of reality inspired Thomas Merton, a Catholic monk, considered to be in stage 6 by Fowler. This faith can motivate belief in the gift of aging from God, which might begin a constructive Christian theology of aging. But this belief has not shaped American public attitudes and policies toward its aging citizens. What is the theology and what are the attitudes that should flow from believing that aging is a gift from God? Public Christianity can supply public meaning to aging and to biomedical ethics. Specifically, we can communicate to the Special Committee on Aging chaired presently (2001) by Senator John Breaux of Louisiana. This committee helps supervise the Health Care Financing Administration, nursing homes, and Medicare. Responsibility for the elderly has gradually shifted from the family to the public with Medicare and Medicaid, and to pastors (Chapter 11) and nurses (Chapter 12).

Chapter 11

Bioethics for Pastors
from a Faith Perspective

As a pastor, I know that pastors need faith too, perhaps even more than the laity. My experience as a pastor is as a campus pastor, a graduate of clinical pastoral education, and a professor of bioethics. Officially, I have served forty-two years with an appointment from my bishop every year. My motivation came from my conversion, a direct encounter with Jesus Christ at age sixteen that transformed me. I became a new person committed to the Kingdom of God on earth. As a consequence of my conversion, even my grades in high school improved enough for me to gain admission to Albion College in Michigan. My campus life there showed me the need for, and the crucial importance of, the campus ministry. In spite of the decline of campus ministry in recent decades, the need exists now more than ever.

Higher education produces the leadership for the future, not only for America but for many other countries. Campus ministry was a frontier movement, especially its ministry with international students. This was face-to-face mission work because the Student Movement was an integral part of the World Student Christian Federation. Many of these international students did return to their home countries to take leadership positions, even cabinet-level positions. Some of our current prominent theologians, such as Lesslie Newbigin, emerged from this encounter between American and international students. But during this early period the number of international students was miniscule compared to today's populations of international students, which are growing exponentially.

During the 1960s, campus ministries were a way to deal academically with the war in Vietnam. The groups included not only international students but also faculty. Thus information was gained from several countries and from experts on the geography, politics, and religion of Vietnam. They compared this information with mainstream media. They tackled in depth an issue, for instance, of whether a humanist claim for conscientious objector status was as legitimate as traditional claims, which were based on religious reasons.

Campus ministry also made major contributions to civil rights. Specifically, we exchanged campus ministries between northern states and Mississippi and other southern states and registered voters who otherwise were prohibited. Our problems of social justice and communication today are equally important, if not even more important. The following is only an outline sketch of some of the problems, our potential response, and the implications of this background for the pastor and bioethics.

PROBLEMS FOR CHRISTIANITY
AND THE UNIVERSITY

A problem from religion: Anti-intellectualism comes from fundamentalism and from our history of revivalism and popular religion, according to Mark Noll (1994) and Richard Hofstadter (1963). Many church clergy search committees do not rank the life of the mind as among the top credentials for being qualified. Another serious concern is raised by Stanley Hauerwas (1994, p. 156) who described the contrast between the selection and attitude of students in the medical school and the divinity school at Duke.

A problem from the university: a significant book, *The Outrageous Idea of Christian Scholarship,* by George Marsden (1997), documents the bias of many academics against the idea that faith leads to learning. The university is "a virtual establishment of nonbelief" according to Marsden. Science is closer to being an established religion, especially if we only consider funding. At the same time, Christian teaching has been privatized. Our culture is therefore hollow, and yet many university search committees are suspicious of degrees in theology and religion.

A problem from the mind: Pluralism reinforces relativism and uncertainty, and America is the most pluralistic country. Ethics, along with religion, has been removed from education in our history. Consequently, history shows religion being used to justify immorality and morality. Therefore, academic (that is, clear and precise) homework is necessary.

To begin, let us note the imperative for the development of the mind from the Old Testament to the New. In Deuteronomy 6:5 (RSV, Oxford Annotated Bible) "You shall love the Lord your God with all your heart, and with all your soul, and with all your might." This is a part of the meaning of the First Commandment in 6:1-25. Next, we note a significant addition, even a fulfillment in Jesus the Christ in Matthew 22:37. "You shall love the Lord your God with all your heart, and with all your soul, and with all your mind" (New American Standard Bible). We need to learn this wisdom and connect it with the functions of church and university, heart and mind, church and seminary, seminary and university.

We also must show the difference that Christian convictions can make. Our one option is to challenge the university with the gospel of faith, hope, and love by dialogue, witness, koinonia, and the transformation that begins with the individual. In Romans 12:2, "Do not be conformed to this world but be transformed by the renewal of your mind, that you may prove what is the will of God." This is a transformation of the mind toward the koinonia calling us and the university to vocation, that is, the church in mission because the world is our parish. This is an academic, rational, moral faith that is needed: "in the world but not of the world." But instead, Stanley Hauerwas (1994) observed that medical students were much more serious about their preparation at Duke than were students preparing for ministry. Also, he contrasted their skills and asked, "What skills and knowledge do ministers have that anyone else does not already have?" (p. 157).

THE NEED FOR AUTHENTIC PROFESSION
IN MINISTRY AND HEALTH CARE

One problem, if not the main problem in bioethics, is that the professions of ministry, medicine, and nursing are marginalized, harassed, and besieged in America. Much authority and trust were lost in the chaos of the 1960s when traditions that supported professions were demeaned and cast aside. The prestige of the ministry declined also with the recession of the mainline denominations and the near-collapse of the campus ministry. It was reported in *The Christian Century* by Religious News Service (1996, p. 39) that academic performance was called into question because 80 percent of applicants were admitted, indicating a lack of quality selection even at Yale Divinity. This criticism was asserted by the other graduate professors at Yale. If Yale Divinity is deficient, what does this mean for the other seminaries? The seminaries at major universities are supposed to be among the best.

Such criticism is extremely damaging because America has given its universities the task of producing competent professionals, especially in the twentieth century. The medical profession responded to this challenge by becoming very successful during the twentieth century. They doubled the life span along with additional extraordinary achievements. If the clergy have not responded in a similar way, what grounds do we have for debating physicians on bioethical issues? Most clergy will probably defend themselves by saying their authority comes from other sources. But the academic community will follow the Yale graduate school authorities and insist that there ought to be common academic standards to be qualified as a professional.

While Yale accepted 80 percent of applicants, there was at the same time an oversupply of clergy. I question the usual definition of oversupply, but we will use it here. Jackson Carroll and Robert Wilson (1980) define and document oversupply in the usual terms that there is a larger number of clergy than churches to be supplied or there is a larger number of newly ordained clergy than the number retiring, again meaning that the supply of ministers exceeds the number of positions for church buildings. One reason I question this definition of oversupply is that it might infer a normative definition of pastor as one who works in a local church. In fact, this is the dominant definition among clergy leaders and laity. This narrow definition tends to undermine the meaning of clergy roles beyond local churches.

The number of clergy in campus ministry, hospital chaplaincy, psychotherapy, and others increased during the oversupply. These pastors specialize in particular competencies of ministry in a manner analogous to specialization in medicine. The difference is that specialization in medicine is recognized as an advancement in competence, in contrast to the clergy where "extended ministries" mean at times the abandonment of ministry. This reality can be illustrated by the frustration of many campus ministers and others who were tired of being asked why they left the ministry.

The oversupply meant a decrease in salaries for clergy. Patricia Chang and Viviana Bompadre (1999, p. 409) note tactfully that earnings affect the prestige of professions, including clergy, and they document that oversupply diminishes professional standing. Many clergy will defend themselves by saying that ministry is not a job because, in contrast, it is a calling. Our pastor reminds our congregation that our problem is that we have too much money. While his warning against materialism is valid, I doubt that he is persuasive on this issue, though he is on most issues. So we need to research fundamental theological questions (along with some scientific ones) about the meaning of profession, vocation, and how we are to be in the world as authentic professionals, and yet not of the world.

Clergy seem unsure that they should become professional. Nevertheless, we are seeing news reports of religious counselors being sued for incompetence. So we need to define effective ministry and discover ways to meet the definition. I offer a general exploratory approach from my dissertation (Hanford, 1974).

DISCERNING THE EFFECTIVENESS OF MINISTRY

There is an urgent need in the seminary, church, and society to detect the qualities of effectiveness of ministry. The major obstacle to solving this problem has been the difficulty, indeed the impossibility thus far, of establishing a valid criterion of effectiveness of ministry. There is a vast literature dealing with this problem. The early literature is well summarized in abstracts by R. J. Menges and J. E. Dittes (1965) in *Psychological Studies of Clergymen*. We will briefly explore this problem, noting the use of the empirical, phenomenological, and synoptic orientations.

Empirical Contribution

A broad empirical approach is basic for solving the problem. Empiricists must continue work on the major obstacle of discovering the criterion of effectiveness. They can engage groups in brainstorming sessions to identify the characteristics of effectiveness. These characteristics can be gleaned from the best surveys of laity, clergy, and representative samples of society. The characteristics would have to be ranked and condensed into a manageable number, perhaps twenty.

Judges could then use these characteristics and select effective ministers, at least 100.

Before accepting this 100 for in-depth study, they would be given psychological tests in an attempt to verify the judges' decisions. Although tests have not so far predicted effectiveness (Douglas, 1957, p. 159), new tests have been constructed and must be used. Douglas' selection of tests was limited to the Rorschach, Strong Vocational Interest Blank, Allport-Vernon Study of Values, and the Cooperative Botany. Milton Rokeach (1960, 1964, 1968, 1969, 1970) has contributed significant studies of values that should be applied to clergy to discover their value systems and to discern their social compassion. These values might be useful for deciding the characteristics of effectiveness. Hiltner and Colston's study (1961) could possibly be applied to evaluate counseling ability. Many instruments from universities could be used to assess teaching competence. The Minnesota Multiphasic Personality Inventory is useful if its results are interpreted along with observations of clergy by well-trained clinicians.

Phenomenological Contribution

The phenomenological approach would challenge the empirical because the two work well when in tension with each other. After the 100 effective clergy were selected by the empirical procedures, the phenomenological approach would be used to further evaluate their characteristics. Douglas (1957, p. 65) discovered that ministers could not accurately estimate their own effectiveness. Therefore the phenomenological approach would not be used for such evaluation but instead for the purpose of facilitating expression from the 100 clergy of the meaning of their characteristics of effectiveness. Through projective techniques, these ministers should be able to disclose additional characteristics of their own. The greatest use of projective techniques with religion is in the clinical effort to screen and counsel ministerial students. These projective techniques have had little development so far in research in religion.

A psychologist of religion could construct open-ended questionnaires for the 100 clergy to express their understanding of their effectiveness and use follow-up questionnaires with in-depth interviews. Guided questions from the survey characteristics could be used to direct these interviews. The psychologist could also meet with the clergy in groups of fifteen for free sharing conversation about the marks of competency and whether they could identify these in one another. These conversations should be recorded and a content analysis made to identify the characteristics of effectiveness. Then these findings could be correlated with the original characteristics. Even though the phenomenological approach lacks validity, it is necessary for gaining insights from the perceptions of the persons who embody the characteristics being sought. The phenomenological approach was slighted in Douglas' study because he could not reveal the case studies of the clergy he worked with. Possibly that material could still be used in some discreet way.

Synoptic Contribution

The main contribution of the synoptic approach is to coordinate the phenomenological and empirical procedures. The researcher would direct them specifically to the problem and devise methods to correlate data, especially as these relate to the characteristics. He or she would review the lives of outstanding clergy, using also psychohistories of effective clergy. Such literature would be scrutinized by content analysis with the characteristics from the survey. Seminary records would be studied, such as application essays. Conference records could also be scrutinized. Maximum validity and reliability would be sought.

An interdisciplinary staff of at least five professionals would be needed to accomplish these comprehensive goals. This complex problem, which is typical in the psychology of religion would require a staff composed of a psychologist of religion as chairperson, a social worker knowledgeable of the ministry, a historian of the ministry, and clinical and educational psychologists with both experience in and knowledge of the ministry.

The synoptic orientation should offer constructive criticism of the other two orientations. Although Douglas' (1957) considerable contribution from limited resources was due to his broad orientation (pp. 166-167), a synoptic orientation is even broader. For example, Douglas limited his view of the ministry primarily to roles. The predominant role, according to both clergy and laity, was that of pastor. Yet the meaning of *pastor* exceeds the category of role. A pastor not only does some function, he is someone special to someone. The latter emphasis requires idiographic research. Douglas found measures of an able or skillful ministry but none of a good minister. The meaning of pastor includes the quality of a good minister.

That the ministry must be understood beyond the institution of the church is a second criticism. Douglas' judges were all church officials. Just as the understanding of religion is diminished when identified with church attendance alone, so is the ministry reduced when identified exclusively with institutional roles. Most persons preparing for ministry do not intend to assume those institutional roles. How are we to discern characteristics for effectiveness for these men and women? John Wesley said the world was his parish. Many contemporary Methodists have taken him seriously and conceive of their ministry as secular. To study the effectiveness of this ministry requires a synoptic view of ministry. There is evidence from studies of campus ministry, for example, which suggests a conflict between effectiveness of campus ministry and compatibility with the traditional church. Douglas also acknowledged the unlikely prospect that prophets would be rated successful in conventional terms.

Last of all, the difficulty of defining the criterion of effectiveness, the major obstacle, certainly requires a synoptic orientation. Empiricists face the danger of reducing the meaning of the criterion to operational terms. Douglas was careful and broad enough to circumvent reductionism, especially of the theological to the psychological alone. Rather than reduce the meaning of effectiveness of ministry, it is wiser to acknowledge that we cannot yet define its effectiveness. We cannot appraise it until we have valid measures. We might also consult Adorno, Frenkel-Brunswik, and Levinson (1950) as an apt model of the synoptic orientation in use, obtaining internal information and establishing validity.

PASTORS AND PHYSICIAN-ASSISTED
SUICIDE OR DEATH

The issue of physician-assisted suicide is fundamentally religious, and pastors are the logical experts on the meaning of religion and death. I will offer examples showing that the issue requires a perspective of informed Christian faith.

The first legalization of assisted death was legislated in the state of Oregon. Religion was identified with fundamentalism and excluded from public debate as a threat to autonomy because of concern that religion would be forced down the throats of Oregonians, according to Courtney Campbell (1999) in *The Christian Century*. A more sophisticated understanding of religion and Christian faith might very well have led to a better decision on this life-or-death issue. The best controlling tool for a humane medical ethic is an informed public motivated by a rational religion such as a public Christianity.

As a second example, during the controversy surrounding Dr. Kevorkian, the function of religion, especially Catholicism, was smeared in public, specifically in Michigan. Much of the fight was between Kevorkian and Right to Life of Michigan. His angry response to their attack was to call religion a medieval force that blocked medical progress. At the same time, he was uncritically swayed by extreme liberal views of religion such as the Unitarian Universalist views of Janet Adkins, the first patient he assisted, in 1990. In 1994 her husband, Ron Adkins, joined in support of Kevorkian as Kevorkian denounced "religious fanatics" and preached, from a Presbyterian church in front of a crucifix, a sermon of autonomy and freedom. By 1996 Kevorkian's firebrand attorney, Geoffrey Fieger, demanded to question prospective jurors for the trial of Kevorkian in order to weed out "religious fanatics." Fieger insisted that the issues were "fundamentally at the heart of religious and moral beliefs" (Associated Press, p. 2). The prosecuting attorney countered that such questioning was against the Constitution's protection of privacy and religious freedom.

Kevorkian's view of autonomy includes his right to condemn religion as medieval and fanatical and to condemn the traditional authority of a physician. Although he talks a lot about patient autonomy, his forceful paternalism and unquestioned physician authority overrides autonomy in his practice of physician-assisted suicide or death.

One of the most perceptive counters to Kevorkian has been offered by physician David Young (1996). When he learned that two-thirds of Catholics in Michigan favored Kevorkian, he wrote his article, which originated from a letter to his bishop, Robert Rose. The substance of his testimony is about his relationship with a ninety-two-year-old patient battling the process of dying. From the mystery of their relationship and of their religion he called upon the Holy Spirit to comfort and free his patient of the struggle. Also, he prayed for the first time. She smiled and died within a short time with her family surrounding her. He was relieved that the dignity of her dying was not compromised by technology. It was a truly sacred religious experience. She was not uncomfortable at the end of life. But I challenge whether anyone ever heard of Dr. Young while we all know that Dr. Kevorkian is a world-renowned celebrity.

Most people with whom I discuss this case see it as a counterargument to Dr. Kevorkian. After closer analysis, this counterpoint is not as obvious as it becomes more clear that this case and the issue about assisted death is extremely difficult and perplexing. It might be clarified further by discussion of relationship, technology versus religion, definition of terminal, active versus passive assisted death, and attitudes toward hospice.

Kevorkian is usually criticized for not having an adequate relationship with the patients he assists. Considering only the one case Young presented, he had three days with the patient before she died. An editor (not named) wrote (Young, 1996) that Young had known the patient in the case for six years. But, I do not know whether Young's relationship was adequate.

Kevorkian obviously used technology. It was apparently effective and he did not charge his patients for remuneration. Was Young's use of religion such as prayer ritual similar to Kevorkian's use of technology? The methods produced basically the same result, namely death. It is possible that Young used medications for pain that shortened the dying process. If true, then Young used technology and probably charged for remuneration.

Kevorkian was appropriately criticized for assisting patients who were not terminal. But, I do not know whether Young's patient was terminal because he did not specify in his case presentation.

Young wrote favorably about hospice. Kevorkian did not maintain favorable work with hospice.

Euthanasia has usually been evaluated on whether the act of killing was active or passive. Kevorkian's use of technology appeared more active than Young's reported action. So the law (stage 4) was against Kevorkian and he remains in jail.

PASTORS AND COMPLEMENTARY
ALTERNATIVE MEDICINE (CAM)

Pastors need to define CAM and clarify its relation to religion and spirituality. "Complementary" usually refers to nonconventional treatments that are used simultaneously with standard Western medicine. "Alternative" means that the nonconventional intervention is used instead of, or in place of, the standard therapy.

CAM is related to spirituality and because spirituality includes so much, it is extremely difficult to define. Adherents of spirituality are known by their frequent affirmation that they are spiritual but not religious. On the other hand, religionists, especially the more orthodox, will claim: I am religious but not spiritual especially when the spiritual is linked with the secular spirituality movement. Harold Koenig (1994, 1997, 1999, and 2001) uses religion and spirituality interchangeably. Most important, Koenig has produced abundant research showing beneficial health effects from both religion and spirituality and his approach could be described not as alternative but rather as complementary medicine.

This tantalizing inquiry cannot be covered in breadth or depth in this small book but I do call for research and discussion by pastors and their communities and others because of concern for health and life, religion and faith. Alternative medicine might be therapeutic but caution is called for if this medicine is used regularly as an alternative to conventional medicine. For example, St. John's wort might help mild depression but will not be adequate to treat cancer.

Decisions about CAM are also relevant to religion and are crucial for America today. Sidney Callahan (1999, p. 57) writes "the spiritual dimension of healing and health provides the alternative perspective of alternate medicine . . . the spirituality of alternative medicine accounts for much of its popular appeal." Alternative medicine has a spiritual background because medicine and religion usually permeate each other in our history and culture. Consider the religious background of psychiatry along with the religious confessional and psychotherapy. Alternative medicine is not only a collection of practices but also core beliefs shaping a metaphysics which attacks conventional medicine's materialism, reliance on instrumental technology. This challenge is empowered by a cultural spirituality, a social movement which includes alternative medicine expressed broadly as holistic medicine, mind over body, spiritual causation of healing, the physics of energy that heals in therapeutic touch as one practice among many.

Well-educated pastors need to work cooperatively with nurses and doctors and also step forth to identify their pastoral expertise to deal with pressing decisions about when CAM is therapeutic and when it is not therapeutic. After all, some of CAM in the form of secular spirituality emerged from religious, even Catholic, sources e.g., Callahan presents. Many parishioners are consumers of CAM. In fact, many are choosing secular spirituality, e.g., transcendental meditation, rather than the Abrahamic religions because of ignorance of the biblical faiths. Knowledgeable interpreters have shown that spirituality is filling a need resulting from the perceived void of meaning in the mainline denominations. Some spirituality advocates have grabbed the power of psychology to create alternative treatments in our culture. Although some parishes are refuting academic psychology, parishioners are embracing spiritual healing, e.g., therapeutic touch, as the equivalent of Christian healing. CAM, as holistic medicine functioning with spiritual causation, is also a challenge, if not a threat, to modern Western scientific medicine. At the same time, some HMOs are selling CAM as an inexpensive and virtuous therapy.

Distinguishing when CAM is therapeutic or healthy and when it is not requires that the competent pastor must have a lay knowledge, at least, of science as a method of knowing. Such a pastor will know the reputable academic journals and read efficacy studies such as the study by John Astin and his colleagues (2000) and Koenig. Since some CAM emerged historically from religious experience, this is pastors' turf and responsibility. Not only sermons but also demanding, rigorous study groups and competent counseling are desperately needed to sort out the harm or benefit of spiritual care, prayer, therapeutic touch, spirituality and evangelism (perhaps in hospitals), meditation on crystals, yoga meditation, Tibetan mysticism, and the power of suggestion in willpower and prayer. Since these matters are frequently in the media, and sometimes sensationalized, the pastoral faith perspective is also needed in this arena of debate and discussion.

But, the contemporary debate can be enlightened by history. Chapter 9 sketched the history of medicine from the nineteenth century into the twentieth. That story included the struggle by mainline medicine to distinguish itself from many alternatives to medicine. Physicians used science and the academic process to mark their identity. Medical schools were evaluated, and their numbers were reduced to include the effective schools. The number of mainline physicians was reduced through a similar process. The American Medical Association was created to provide an institution for effective professionals to continue the process. This history continues today by scrutinizing CAM. Nurses and pastors need a similar model. Pastors need to distinguish alternative spirituality from mainline religion to show authentic, healthy religion. Much of alternative spirituality can be integrated into traditional mainline religion and much of alternative medicine can be integrated into conventional medicine.

THE PASTOR AND THE CONSENT PROCEDURE

Since a pastor is in direct contact with patients and their families, the pastor can facilitate the consent procedure about treatments in health care. A family needs to be united in agreement on consent. Organ donation, for instance, is often blocked because the family of a potential donor has not been informed of the patient's decision to donate. The following guidelines can help the process of consent and create a therapeutic relationship.

1. Know the characteristics of a moral practitioner-patient relationship, such as a stage 5 and/or 6 model of contract-covenant relationship.
2. The patient almost always has the right to informed consent.
3. Research shows that patients want complete information even when the information is anxiety producing.
4. The patient decides when the information is complete.
5. The proxy or advocate gives consent when the patient is not competent, as when the patient is a fetus or a child, in which case the parents usually give the substitute consent.
6. When an adult is unconscious or irrational, the proxy might be the spouse, next of kin, court, or other advocate.
7. The test for a valid substitute consent is whether such consent represents the best interest of the patient. If parents do not represent the child's best interest, then the state is obligated to do so.
8. The practitioner is the authority for technical information.
9. The patient is the authority for ethical decisions.
10. The practitioner might nevertheless facilitate ethical decisions by the patient.
11. Hospital ethics committees often assist communication between the practitioner and patient and others for difficult decisions.

12. The practitioner has the right of conscience not to participate, for example, in abortions, but is still obligated to care for example, by giving a referral.
13. The consent form represents the right of consent, autonomy, and freedom of the patient.
14. The Patients' Bill of Rights of 1972 includes many of these points and implies correlate duties of practitioners. For example, when patients have the right to information, then practitioners have the duty to disclose or give the information for a meaningful transparent consent. Transparent communication has so much light shining through it that one easily sees through because of the honesty and clarity.
15. Trust is necessary for effective practice.

If these guidelines are applied in practice, malpractice suits are less likely.

Additional rights or responsibilities will contribute to the fiduciary covenant. The health practitioner also has rights, so the patient has a duty to be honest and sincere. The very important SUPPORT study (The SUPPORT Principal Investigators, 1995) taught us to beware of routine procedures.

This massive empirical study over five years showed that physicians could be so engrossed in the habits of rapid, routine practice that routine procedures were done without consent from elders who were subjects in the study. This preoccupation with technological procedures caused harm and unnecessary pain and suffering to these elders. Even after specialized nurses were employed to assist the communication necessary for consent, the routine continued for several years.

To be well informed with accurate information for consent, I believe patients should own their medical records. In fact, I beg our hospital leaders, one of whom is a former student of mine, to please send the results of my laboratory tests to me, because it was my blood and money that produced the tests. Consent is not authentic without information, and therefore patients need access to their records. When my mother was very ill in her last years, she would complain to me about her doctor after her appointments. We eventually confronted this problem, and her physician of many years agreed to give her records to us when we arrived to wait for her appointment. With managed care, the average time for an appointment is only seven minutes, so the patient must be well informed to benefit from a brief office visit.

Because of the abuses to patients in health maintenance organizations, we need a new Bill of Rights to update the old bill of 1972. The new bill specifically would give patients the power to sue HMOs. Unfortunately, the Supreme Court voted against the patient in the important case, *Herdrich vs. Pegram.* The duty or responsibility for patients' rights is now in the Congress, which means the ultimate responsibility lies with an informed citizenry.

CONCLUSION

We need pastors to interpret bioethics from their faith perspective. Now that bioethics is in its third period of historical development, according to Renee Fox (1994), the prophetic imperative of the public religion and church is needed especially and is very relevant. We need to combine our emphasis on personal virtue, which Stanley Hauerwas emphasizes, and public justice, which Courtney Campbell discusses with his emphasis on prophetic religion.

This balance can also contribute to developing an effective professional ministry. In addition, I recommend accepting the challenge from Yale to advance the academic and scientific dimensions of a professional ministry along with the theological and biblical.

The pastor's interpretation needs to be academically sound and biblical. To be academically sound, we go to the university to seek understanding. But there we might not find Christian understanding, and even discover that Christian scholarship is not allowed. We need the gospel good news proclaimed to the mind so we can love and serve with our mind and heart.

How are we to love God with all our mind when we cannot find any genuine secure certainty? We venture forth with our Bible and the scientific method. Christian religion without science lacks a method for new understanding. Science without religion lacks a source for deep understanding and meaning. William James (1902, 1961), in *The Varieties of Religious Experience,* suggested that theology must give way to a "science of religions." Today a public theology requires a broad view of science for a Christian religion that makes meaning public. The Christian Coalition has a narrow view of Christianity and of public life, especially public political life. Thus the public church must be an authentic church or the church in its own right defined by its canon and yet sensitive to its mission in and toward a public order. This is the church called to be the parent of each Christian and perhaps in our day, the responsible Christian who forges a credible faith personally and in witness to others.

This church will inform its families of the essentials of bioethics, enabling them to know a good practitioner-client relationship, including their rights and consent procedures, and will project a faith perspective into bioethics.

The pastor is needed to illuminate the theological and clinical dimensions of major issues in medical ethics and thereby develop a responsible church and an informed citizenry to create a caring society. There is a bright future for pastors and for public religion to deal with the serious problems of biomedical ethics. Public religion is social religion. Since medicine is increasingly a corporate enterprise, the religious critic, pastor, or public theologian must enter public debate on managed care, insurance company power, and politics. A book by R. DeVries and J. Subedi (1998), *Bioethics and Society,* includes additional suggestions for further research by sociologists of religion to forge a public religion for bioethics in the twenty-first century by pastors and by nurses (see Chapter 12).

Chapter 12

Bioethics for Nurses
from a Faith Perspective

This chapter for nurses offers an opportunity for a brief summary of the book, and the summary serves as an introduction to this chapter. Nurses are the largest group of health practitioners, and they are central to bioethics because they are literally in the middle of the relationship between the patient and the doctor. The nurse usually spends the most time within this relationship. Chapter 1 focused on nursing students in my research using Kohlberg, and nurses have researched more on the Kohlberg method, stages, and literature than any other health profession. Their curriculum often includes Erik Erikson's development of personality and Kohlberg's view of personality followed by his strong emphasis on cognitive development along with attention to emotion, especially within the early stages. Fowler's work is known by the large number of nurses who have profound religious faith commitments. Many Catholic nurses are interested in Kohlberg, probably because Jesuits were attracted to Kohlberg's emphasis on logic and natural law. Fowler taught at Boston College, a prestigious Catholic institution, and his work is attractive to both Catholic and Protestant nurses, including those in the Reformed tradition. Nurses typically embody in their personhood and profession the meaning of the therapeutic relationship as discussed in Chapter 4. In fact, many of them are now considering identifying their role and profession mainly with caring even over curing (which might be preferred by physicians).

Nurses were powerfully impacted and threatened by the early struggles with the managed care system, which was discussed in Chapter 7. Nurses are the key health professionals in considering organ donation (Chapter 6). Through e-mails and the Internet, I have observed strong interest and expertise among nurses about genetics and counseling

(Chapter 8). For example, I will summarize the new opportunities for nurses to become competent to deliver care in the use of genetics for diagnosis, genetic counseling, and new treatments from the advances in genetic research. Gwen Anderson (RN, PhD) of Stanford University is a leader in this endeavor. She will offer courses on these topics.

As with the physicians discussed in Chapter 9, nurses also struggle with the machines of technology at the bedside, and they are the main source of care for the elderly (Chapter 10). Even in relation to pastoral care (Chapter 11), nurses are working with pastors in a growing movement practicing effective care in the parish setting.

In this last chapter, I describe the struggle and progress by nurses, who are becoming more professional, including a representative nurse who embodies a faith perspective.

IS THE NURSE A PROFESSIONAL?

What I said about the importance of professionalism for clergy and physicians in Chapter 11 is even more crucial for nurses. Their main challenge for the twenty-first century is to establish the integrity and solidarity of their profession. Presently, they are viewed as a quasi-profession, which is somewhat similar to the predicament of clergy described in Chapter 11. Nurses are perceived as having half of a profession because they have a clear and well thought-out code of ethics and they fulfill the service or altruistic dimension of authentic professionalism. Again, these requirements are also met by clergy in their effort to be considered a profession.

Both professions, nevertheless, need the model of the American Medical Association to complete the other half of the requirements to be recognized as a bona fide profession. Since about 1900, the AMA has united and standardized their profession by setting forth rigorous demands for higher education. Nurses have not taken charge or control of their profession and have not set forth academic demands similar to those of physicians. Appropriate requirements for nurses are careful selection of students, a standard degree, and research. These are necessary to become fully professional.

Managed care will force nurses (and physicians) into its corporate mold if nurses do not take control of their profession. When managed care relies exclusively on the bottom line, it destroys the needed discretion and trust of the nurses and doctors. These are professional qualities that must be maintained if quality care is to be delivered. Patients fear that the one who pays the bill will decide what necessary treatment is. Actually, patients provide the payment by paying the premiums for their insurance coverage. This point must be emphasized to counter the notion that the HMO and the employer are paying the bill. Employees often must take a salary cut to contract for health insurance. The American public must deal with the fact that the insurance industry not only does not actually pay the bill but takes 25 percent of the financial resources for its own operation and delivers no health care itself. Thus, health professionals need to be supported when they assert their distinctive leadership in defining the therapeutic relationship and exercising their necessary control within the health system.

When I wrote my research report, summarized in Chapter 1, about advancing moral reasoning with nursing students, my long-range goal was to contribute to excellence in clinical practice, which has always been the mark of the competent professional nurse. Such competence includes both technical and ethical competence. This research on moral and faith development has progressed from moral reasoning to building a bridge from moral thinking to moral action, culminating in professional nursing practice.

Laura Ducket and Muriel Ryden (1994) and James Rest (1994, 1998, p. 59, 1999) show a .58 correlation between scores on the Defining Issues Test and clinical performance. The earlier research by Sheehan and colleagues (1980) on doctors also supports this finding. The DIT is a multiple-choice test measuring the moral reasoning of the test-taker who analyzes and evaluates the most important considerations when thinking through a moral dilemma. A moral dilemma presents a conflict in moral thinking about an issue and about what standards for moral evaluation should be used. The student's selection of items from the test indicates the developmental level of moral reasoning. Further description of my own use of the instrument is summarized in Chapter 1.

Researchers at the University of Minnesota have identified the steps for learning ethics that lead toward ethical professional practice. They have identified a body of moral knowledge, including who should teach this curriculum, how it should be taught, and how to implement a moral decision in nursing practice. Here the ethics of teaching is integrated into clinical practice, and the quality of the clinical practice is evaluated by a clinical professor with a clinical evaluation tool that assesses performance. These measuring instruments are studied to establish their reliability and validity. The results, especially on the DIT, are so impressive that the nursing school and others are tempted to use its findings for assisting in the selection of students. Three of four groups of nursing students demonstrated significant advancement in moral reasoning from pre- and post-tests of scores on the DIT. Thus, much progress has been achieved by empirical academic work toward establishing technical and ethical professional competence.

The worst damage to a profession occurs when it is sold in the cheapest manner. For example, when a physician, hospital, or HMO hires the least trained or least educated nurse for the lowest salary, the demand for professional excellence is destroyed. Most professionals have not been overtrained so much as their professional function has not been understood or appreciated.

Many additional problems concern the American Nurses Association (ANA). Hospital staffing practices are unsafe because nurses are regularly forced to work long hours with excessive overtime. New York nurses have protested this staffing issue by picketing. The management of Southside Hospital in New York initially refused to address the staffing problem. But nevertheless, the 400 nurses at the Nyack Hospital won their struggle. They created a strong consensus and signed a five-year contract that includes language to ensure safe staffing and improvement of working conditions (NursingInsider, May 25, 2000).

The United American Nurses (UAN) organized their National Labor Assembly on June 21, 2000 to prepare nationally for present and future labor disputes. The UAN will provide a strong labor voice for the ANA, develop leadership, assist in bargaining, and strengthen further the UAN and the ANA. To gain power, they are continuing affiliation talks with the AFL-CIO.

I sincerely hope that all these efforts will succeed, because the nurses' claims, especially for safety and staffing, are justified by the principle of justice. From my painful, even traumatic experience of three strikes, I have observed that the strike is a limited and questionable strategy as a protest action. To win, such action must gain political support from citizens generally, and many of them will feel hurt by the strike. Presently, America does not seem to accept the justice claims and does not give decisive support. The political mood is more negative than positive toward unions and is even more intensely negative toward strikes.

Consequently, the ANA is wise in beefing up its development of an authentic profession by increasing demands for education and bona fide academic degrees along with advancing serious research. They have produced research, most notably at the University of Minnesota under the outstanding leadership of the late James Rest, showing the correlation between moral reasoning and moral and competent clinical performance. Complementing this research on ethics, nurses are advancing their research also in more technical areas of practice.

In addition, nurses are mounting a major offensive in response to the damaging effects of managed care. I elaborated the damaging effects on mental health practitioners in Chapter 7, and I point to the nurses' own critical response here. In 1994, nurses, predominantly those associated with managed health care, organized The American Association of Managed Care Nurses (<http://www.aamcn.org>). This professional group is defining standards for managed care nursing, educating nurses with critical thinking skills, and learning specifics about managed care. They produce resources, specifically *The Journal of Managed Care Medicine* and their textbook, *A Nurse's Introduction to Managed Care* (American Association of Managed Care Nurses, 2000).

These sources guide and connect two roles in nursing, direct patient care and administration of nursing practice. They plan to inform and impact public policy in support of their mission. To implement this national organization, state chapters are being established from Florida to Nevada, including Washington, DC. With these efforts, nurses are asserting their power of professional ethical values to regulate a market that controls managed care. They step up against the bottom line, including exorbitant salaries for CEOs in managed care corporations, which also take higher profits than other business groups. Frequently, in opposition to such forces of commodification or commercialism, nurses must make independent professional judgments about a patient's clinical condition from within a therapeutic relationship between a particular nurse, doctor, and patient.

Eliot Freidson (1990), a distinguished sociologist of medicine, documents the centrality of professionalism to health care. The professional must be motivated by the quality performance of practice enunciated by the special knowledge of professionals and supported by their own community of solidarity, who will also stimulate the courage to make discretionary judgments for the patient. This will create and enhance the patient's trust, which is necessary for healing.

Many expert critics of managed care insist that universal health care is the solution to "mangled" health systems. For example, the president of the American Nurses Association, Mary Foley, has offered a proposal for universal coverage for health care. Specifically, she recommends that Medicare become universal. She argues that Medicare is American, is successful, and can be expanded to cover the American population including parity for coverage of those suffering with mental illness (CSPAN, January 20, 2000).

FAITH PERSPECTIVE

Many nurses embody a faith perspective including Christian faith. One current representative is Judith Shelly, an RN with a doctorate in ministry, who is director of resources for Nurses Christian Fellowship and editor of the *Journal of Christian Nursing*. Most of all, she captures the Christian faith perspective on death as the last enemy (I Corinthians 15:22-26). The thrust of Western medical history seems to show that the faith commitment to battle death has motivated the development of medicine and nursing in the West and especially here in America. This Christian conviction accepts the tragedy of death, that is, the crucifixion precedes the resurrection. Jesus did in fact suffer death on the cross. The dominant metaphors for Western practitioners have been military metaphors such as to battle death, write orders, and command younger practitioners in their training and discipline. Florence Nightingale launched nursing on a military mission.

In contrast, the East has generally accepted death as a passing of the seasons, therefore without the tragic dimension. Consequently, there has been less intense commitment to aggressive treatment and development of medical institutions in the East.

Elizabeth Kübler-Ross has apparently been influenced by Eastern thought, and she has impacted nursing in America. Some studies of American nurses have shown a decline in their commitment to the sanctity of life principle in the sense that this standard required fighting death. Such trends produced concern that Dr. Kübler-Ross's influence might create a chasm between nurses and physicians who embody the traditional combat against death. Ross spoke on our campus several times, and I noticed large numbers of nurses in the audience but rarely a physician.

If this is true, then we need to be reminded of our valuable tradition by nurse Shelly (Shelly and Miller, 1999, p. 190) who confronts the horror of death. The Bible hints at a natural death in Genesis 25:8. But she does not accept "natural" as a categorical virtue word. Often the natural requires intervention. In fact, intervention is much of what the medical and nursing practice do. They intervene before the natural process leads to death and suffering. Death separates us from our loved ones. This faith perspective on the reality of death is from Christianity. Shelly integrates her faith into her professional practice, and this makes a difference in favor of life over death. Her faith and hope in the resurrection can empower her for the demanding, strenuous struggle against disease, pain, and death. She accepts the survey of Christian nurses, 80 percent of whom ranked compassion as the top characteristic of a good nurse along with competence, faith, integrity, and responsibility. Here we can see why nurses are often and traditionally looked up to since they are considered to be the conscience of health practitioners. Notice the word "science" in "conscience." The word means knowing with, that is, to know what is right from universal moral principles and a faith perspective.

DOES FAITH CONTRIBUTE
TO EFFECTIVE PRACTICE?

Shelly's (Shelly and Miller, 1999) faith perspective leads toward effective practice because her view of Christian faith includes a moral imperative to serve, just as Florence Nightingale sought to join faith with ethics and service. Shelly's emphasis on compassion can be interpreted as suffering with or feeling with the patient and using empathy (defined and discussed in Chapter 1) to communicate at a deep level. She stresses and insists that competence must include the best science, technology, and the development of specific nursing skills. Her faith is not blind but is accountable to truth in the history of Christianity, in her self-aware conscience, and in her respect for science. She does not shy away from power but seeks its source, does critical evaluation, and decides whether power comes from authentic faith.

Finally, she counts on results that can be known, understood, accepted by other capable health professionals, and in harmony with healing in the Bible.

CONCLUSION

This chapter is an advocacy of nursing because nurses are the consistent advocates for caring for the patient. Suggestions were offered to embodying this caring in solid professional structures of academic excellence, rigorous research, and responsible political action for justice and for the integrity of the profession. With such commitment to authentic professionalism and a faith perspective, there can be victory over death, pain, and suffering through the effective practice of nursing.

Conclusion

Two perspectives and five objectives have guided and now summarize the construction of this book. The first perspective is from a broad yet decisive understanding of Christian faith, which is not intended to be exclusive but inclusive and in dialogue with the many other perspectives of our pluralistic society. This faith perspective I have shown to be compatible with the scientific method. The second perspective is indispensable for studying and doing or practicing bioethics. Science is about knowing and can be defined by its method. This view must not be confused with scientism, which functions almost as a quasi religion and tends to reduce the substance of Christianity and other such perspectives. Both Christian faith and the methods of science can be self-correcting, that is, they can help us cut through self-deception and illusion. That must be our first task before offering guidance for bioethics.

Throughout this book I have concentrated on the first of five objectives, listed in the introduction. I emphasized specifically the importance and meaning of the technical-ethical distinction. To do bioethics, we must know and identify the moral domain to know the moral problem. Otherwise, ethics is glossed over and not identified, leaving all the focus and discussion on the technical. For example, the main case in Chapter 4 presented a physician conscientiously carrying out his routine of technical repair of the body of a patient who wanted to die. They never settled the ethical controversy concerning consent by the patient. The result was that nothing truly therapeutic ever happened because the fundamental ethical necessity of consent and contract were never added to a working relationship between the physician and the patient with Lou Gehrig's disease. Thus our first objective was and is to be clear about the distinction between the technical and ethical, especially in practice. For example, evaluating side effects and best treatment are technical issues within the appropriate authority of the physicians, which answers the ethical question about who is to decide. Of course, patients still have a right to refuse treatment. But once again, if this issue goes to court, the precedent and guideline is that the court will decide with the legal and moral standard, namely, what is in the best interests of the patient? We can predict that the court, that is the judge, will decide to meet the demand that best interests requires, especially in a decision that orders treatment with the greatest probability for life.

To achieve the second objective, I offered a rational framework in the form of moral philosophical principles, especially in Chapter 1 and Christian faith viewpoints throughout the book. The Protestant convictions of Fowler and the classic Catholic commitments of Pellegrino were presented in some detail. Then, application or interpretation of these stances and others were elaborated. Since the self is inevitably involved in this inquiry, insights from developmental psychology were integrated with theology, especially in the chapters on Fowler and several others.

To achieve the third objective, I stressed the crucial significance of the quality of the therapeutic relationship between practitioner and patient throughout the book. Faith is necessary but perhaps not sufficient to build trust (which is often missing) in the relationship. Obviously the practitioner must add competence to the relationship. Therefore the purpose of teaching bioethics is to enhance the development of technical *and* ethical practitioners and responsible clients. The quality of the relationship increases, if not decides, therapeutic effectiveness. Christian agape (a Greek word for love as active concern) can provide the therapeutic healing and motivation for caring in health care. Technology enhances good and effective treatment if it does not become a substitute for a quality relationship, as articulated in Chapter 9 and elsewhere. For instance, psychiatric medicines have brought wondrous results, especially when accompanied by a caring and guiding relationship.

All three objectives lead toward a Christian therapeutic bioethics. The fourth objective projects a standard to discern: when are medicine, bioethics, and Christian faith therapeutic? In Chapter 4, Pellegrino insisted that medicine is therapeutic when it practices both curing and caring. Such practice requires that the practitioner must be technically competent for curing and ethically competent for genuine caring. The major study in the *Journal of the American Medical Association* (The SUPPORT Principal Investigators, 1995) showed that some physicians knew what was moral, but they did not practice what was moral. Frequently, consent was not obtained, patients were treated aggressively against their will, and suffering resulted. Some doctors followed their routine regardless of the patient's wishes. Other practitioners followed their view of the legal more than what was moral.

I advocate a Christian faith to fill the gap between knowing and doing, described briefly here and throughout this text, especially in Chapter 4. Also, in Chapters 2 and 3, I summarized Fowler's empirical evidence that Christian faith motivates us to be moral and to act morally. His interpretation of the advancement from stage 4 to stage 5 faith, which embodies a mature use of cognitive and emotional meaning in Christian faith. In this way, bioethics is therapeutic when it translates such moral faith into practice. In spite of the death of James Rest, his researchers at the University of Minnesota are showing that moral faith can be translated into practice, and they even show how this can be done. Fowler's ongoing research in pastoral care through the public church also contributes to the pioneering work of creating a therapeutic Christian bioethics.

The fifth and final objective demands a summary case analysis along with the many other cases throughout this book, because these show how we can practice bioethics. Since the overall thrust of this work has highlighted the significance of thinking comprehensively about bioethics from a faith perspective, the following case will show that Christian faith can and frequently does make a therapeutic difference in bioethics.

I have chosen a very controversial case, the Helga Wanglie story (Levine, 1997). Mrs. Wanglie, an eighty-five-year-old patient, was taken from her nursing home for emergency treatment of shortness of breath and to widen her breathing passages on January 1, 1990. Her condition worsened, and she was connected to a respirator. Later there were efforts to wean her from the respirator, but these efforts failed. Her heart stopped; she was resuscitated and taken to intensive care. Since she remained unconscious, a physician suggested withdrawal of life support. Later other physicians concluded that she was in a persistent vegetative state and also suggested withdrawal of the respirator. Costs were mounting to $700,000. But the family insisted that her last consent was for aggressive treatment drawn from her Christian faith and hope.

To demonstrate the intensity of conflicting views in her story, here is a brief historical sketch. During the 1980s, momentum grew in America in support of the right to die, especially with the publicity given to Dr. Jack Kevorkian. During the 1990s, the Wanglie advocates argued strenuously in the opposite direction, because the powerful convictions of their evangelical Christian faith united the family and empowered the father, Oliver Wanglie, who was also an attorney. Therefore, he was well equipped for the struggle. Let us begin with definitions and later consider Wanglie's argument.

The definition of futility appears to be technical at first sight. On a second look, the definition is extremely vague and becomes dependent on who is defining. Here, the physician using a narrow definition of futility runs the risk of imposing not only his or her technical judgment but also an ethical judgment. Since knowing whether someone might recover from a prevegetative state is almost impossible, the physician might be influenced by a responsibility to contain cost. On the other hand, the patient might be guided by strong faith and hope. Whose value judgment should prevail? This relates to the ethical and religious liberty in the Constitution, a stage 6 principle according to Lawrence Kohlberg and James Fowler. A claim for religious liberty is also supported in the Helga Wanglie case. In addition, the physician uses a narrow definition of futility and runs the risk of playing God. Perhaps only God knows when a patient might emerge conscious from a prevegetative state.

The father remained firm and steadfast. At the end of his major struggle he affirmed, "We felt that when she was ready to go that the good Lord would call her, and I would say that was what happened" (Levine, 1997, p. 131). The struggle pitted the Wanglies against powerfully authoritative, well-informed, and ethical physicians and against a national attitude that was increasingly favorable toward managed care. The Wanglies supported and reinforced their faith perspective by adding widely accepted moral guidelines such as the almost absolute right of consent by the patient, as in the Patients' Bill of Rights (American Hospital Association, 1972). Helga had clearly told her husband that she did not want her life shortened. He became increasingly her legal and faithful surrogate, with the united support of their family.

I believe evidence shows that the Christian faith of this family influenced, if not determined, and certainly strengthened their position, which was confirmed by a court. I am not arguing simply for the content of this decision but also for the form and content of a Christian faith perspective along with reason, logic, and moral philosophy and theology. (Form and content were defined in Chapter 2.) That faith perspective did and will make a difference.

References

Introduction

Barbour, I. (1993). *Ethics in an Age of Technology.* San Francisco: Harper.
Callahan, D. (1990). Religion and the secularization of bioethics. *Hastings Center Report, 20*(July), 2-4.
Fletcher, J. (1954). *Morals and Medicine.* Princeton, NJ: Princeton University Press.
Marty, M. (1990). *Healthy People 2000: A Role for America's Religious Communities.* Chicago: The Carter and Park Ridge Centers.
Palmer, P. (1981). *The Company of Strangers.* New York: Crossroads.
Pence, G. (1990). *Classic Cases in Medical Ethics.* New York: McGraw-Hill.
Ramsey, P. (1970). *The Patient As Person.* New Haven, CT: Yale University Press.
Siegler, M. (1991). The secularization of medical ethics. *Update, 7*(July), 1-8.
Tubbs, J. (1990). *Recent Theological Approaches in Medical Ethics.* Unpublished doctoral dissertation, University of Virginia.

Chapter 1

Beck, C. (1972). *Stimulating Transition to Post-Conventional Morality: The Pickering High School Study.* Toronto: Ontario Institute for Studies in Education.
Boyd, D.R. (1976). *Education Toward Principled Moral Judgment: An Analysis of an Experimental Course in Undergraduate Moral Education Applying Lawrence Kohlberg's Theory of Moral Development.* Unpublished EdD dissertation, Harvard University.
Everding, H., Wilcox, M.M., Huffaker, L.A., and Snelling, C.H. (1998). *Viewpoints.* Harrisburg, PA: Trinity Press.
Fowler, J. (1981). *Stages of Faith.* San Francisco: Harper and Row.
Koenig, H. (1999). *The Healing Power of Faith.* New York: Simon and Schuster.
Kohlberg, L. (1981). *Essays on Moral Development.* Volume 1: *The Philosophy of Moral Development.* New York: Harper and Row.
Kohlberg, L. (1984). *Essays on Moral Development.* Volume 2: *The Psychology of Moral Development.* San Francisco: Harper and Row.
Lawrence, J. (1987). Verbal processing of the Defining Issues Test by principled and non-principled moral reasoners. *Journal of Moral Education, 16*(2), 117-130.
Martin, R.M., Shafto, M., and Vandeinse, W. (1977). The reliability, validity, and design of the Defining Issues Test. *Developmental Psychology, 13*(5), 460-468.

Niebuhr, R. (1943). *The Nature and Destiny of Man.* New York: Charles Scribner's Sons.

Rest, J. (1986). *Moral Development.* New York: Praeger.

Rest, J. (1994). *Moral Development in the Professions.* Hillsdale, NJ: Erlbaum.

Rest, J. (1999). *Post-Conventional Moral Thinking: A Neo-Kohlbergian Approach.* Hillsdale, NJ: Erlbaum.

Self, D. (1994). Moral reasoning in medicine. In J. Rest (Ed.) *Moral Development in the Professions.* Hillsdale, NJ: Erlbaum.

Sheehan, T.J., Husted, S.D., Candee, D., Cook, C.D., and Bargen, M. (1980). Moral judgment as a predictor of clinical performance. *Evaluation and the Health Professions, 3*(4), 393-404.

Tillich, P. (1957). *Dynamics of Faith.* New York: Harper and Brothers Publishers.

Chapter 2

Fowler, J. (1974). Faith, liberation, and human development. *The Foundation, 79,* 1-30.

Fowler, J. (1976). Stages in faith: The structural-developmental approach. In T. Hennessy (Ed.), *Values and Moral Development* (pp. 173-210). New York: Paulist Press.

Fowler, J. (1978). Life-faith patterns: Structures of trust and loyalty. In J. Berryman (Ed.), *Life Maps: Conversations on the Journey of Faith* (pp. 14-101). Minneapolis: Winston Press.

Fowler, J. (1989). Faith and belief. In R. Hunter (Ed.), *Dictionary of Pastoral Care* (pp. 1-10). Nashville, TN: Abingdon Press.

Fowler, J. (1996). *Faithful Change.* Nashville, TN: Abingdon Press.

Greenawalt, K. (1988). *Religious Convictions and Political Choice.* New York: Oxford University Press.

Hauerwas, S. (1997). *Wilderness Wandering.* Boulder, CO: Westview Press.

Kohlberg, L. (1967). Moral and religious education and the public schools. In T. Sizer (Ed.), *Religion and Public Education.* Boston: Houghton Mifflin.

Kohlberg, L. (1974). Education, moral development and faith. *Journal of Moral Education 4*(1), 5-16.

Kohlberg, L. (1981). *Essays on Moral Deveolpment.* New York: Harper and Row.

Kohlberg, L. (1982). A reply to Owen Flanagan. *Ethics 92*(3), 516.

Marty, M. (1991). How to draw guidance from a heritage. In B. Kogan (Ed.), *A Time to Be Born* (pp. 241-256). New York: Walter de Gruyter.

Parks, S. (1990). Faith development in a changing world. *The Drew Gateway 60*(1) pp. 4-21.

Power, F.C. and Kohlberg, L. (1980). Religion, morality, and ego development. In C. Brusslemans (Ed.), *Toward Moral and Religious Maturity* (pp. 51-85). Morristown, NJ: Silver Burdette.

Shulik, R. (1979). *Faith Development, Moral Development*. Unpublished doctoral dissertation, University of Chicago, Chicago.

Snarey, J. (1991). Faith development, moral development, and nontheistic Judaism: A construct validity study. In W. Kurtines and J. Gewirtz (Eds.), *Handbook of Moral Behavior and Development* (p. 303). Hillsdale, NJ: Erlbaum.

Thiemann, R. (1996). *Religion in Public Life.* Washington, DC: Georgetown.

Chapter 3

Avery, W. (1990). A Lutheran examines James W. Fowler. *Religious Education, 85* (1), 69-83.

Fernhout, J. (1986). Where is faith: Searching for the core of the cube. In C. Dykstra and S. Parks (Eds.), *Faith Development and Fowler* (pp. 65-89). Birmingham, AL: Religious Education Press.

Fowler, J. (1978). Life/faith patterns: Structures of trust and loyalty. In J. Berryman (Ed.), *Life Maps: Conversations on the Journey of Faith* (pp. 14-101), Minneapolis: Winston Press.

Fowler, J. (1981). *Stages of Faith: The Psychology of Human Development and the Quest for Meaning.* New York: Harper and Row.

Fowler, J. (1983). Practical theology and the shaping of Christian lives. In D. Browning (Ed.), *Practical Theology* (pp. 148-166). San Francisco: Harper.

Fowler, J. (1984). *Becoming Adult, Becoming Christian.* New York: Harper and Row.

Fowler, J. (1986a). Dialogue toward a future. In C. Dykstra and S. Parks (Eds.), *Faith Development and Fowler* (pp. 275-301). Birmingham, AL: Religious Education Press.

Fowler, J. (1986b). Faith and the structuring of meaning. In C. Dykstra and S. Parks (Eds.), *Faith Development and Fowler* (pp. 15-44). Birmingham, AL: Religious Education Press.

Fowler, J. (1987). *Faith Development and Pastoral Care.* Philadelphia: Fortress Press.

Fowler, J. (1988). The public church and Christian nurture. In K. Nipkow and F. Schweitzer (Eds.), *Stages of Faith and Religious Development* (p. 12 refers to Fowler's chapter, pp. 1-19, which was published in the German edition of this book). New York: Crossroad.

Fowler, J. (1990). Faith/belief. In R.J. Hunter (Ed.), *Dictionary of Pastoral Care and Counseling* (pp. 394-397). Nashville: Abingdon Press.

Fowler, J. (1991). *Weaving the New Creation: Stages of Faith and the Public Church.* New York: Harper.

Hanford, J. (1975). A synoptic approach: Resolving problems in empirical and phenomenological approaches to the psychology of religion. *Journal for the Scientific Study of Religion, 14* (3), 219-228.

Hanford, J. (1982). Book review. *Journal for the Scientifc Study of Religion, 21* (4), 383-384.

Kohlberg, L. (1984). *Essays on Moral Development.* San Francisco: Harper and Row.

Malony, H. (1990). The concept of faith in psychology. In J. Lee (Ed.), *Handbook of Faith* (pp. 71-98). Birmingham, AL: Religious Education Press.

McDargh, J. (1984). Faith development theory at ten years. *Religious Studies Review, 10* (4), 339-343.

Moseley, R. (1991). Forms of logic in faith development theory. *Pastoral Psychology,* 39 (3), 143-152.

Oosterhuis, A. (1989). On de-staging our relationships. *Journal of Psychology and Theology, 17* (1), 16-20.

Osmer, R. (1990). James Fowler and the reformed tradition: An exercise in theological reflection in religious education. *Religious Education, 85* (1), 51-68.

Rest, J. (1999). Postconventional Moral Thinking. Hillsdale, NJ: Erlbaum.

Snarey, J. (1991). Faith development. In W. Kurtines (Ed.), *Handbook of Moral Behavior* (pp. 279-306). Hillsdale, NJ: Erlbaum.

Streib-Weickum, H. (1989). *Hermeneutics of Metaphor, Symbol, and Narrative in Faith Development Theory.* Doctoral dissertation, Emory University.

Tracy, D. (1975). *Blessed Rage for Order.* New York: Crossroad-Seabury Books.

Tracy, D. (1981). *The Analogical Imagination.* New York: Crossroad.

Tracy, D. (1987). *Plurality and Ambiguity.* San Francisco: Harper and Row.

Wuthnow, R. (1982). A sociological perspective. In K. Stokes (Ed.), *Faith Development in the Adult Life Cycle* (pp. 209-224). New York: Sadlier.

Chapter 4

Hastings Center Report, Special Supplement. "Dying Well in the Hospital: The Lessons of SUPPORT." 25(November-December) 1995: s1-s48.

Macklin, R. (1993). *Enemies of Patients.* New York: Oxford University Press.

Pellegrino, E. (1985). The caring ethic. In A.H. Bishop and J.R. Scudder Jr. (Eds.), *Caring, Curing, Coping* (pp. 8-30). Alabama: University of Alabama Press.

Pellegrino, E. and Thomasma, D. (1993). *The Virtues in Medical Practice.* New York: Oxford University Press.

The Right to Die. VHS, 20 minutes. Carle Medical Communications. Urbana, Illinois, 1985.

The SUPPORT Principal Investigators. (1995). A controlled trial to improve care for seriously ill hospitalized patients. *Journal of the American Medical Association, 274*(20), 1591-1598.

Chapter 5

Siegler, M. (1991). The secularization of medical ethic. *Update,* (2)7(June), 1-8.

Siegler, M., Pellegrino, E., and Singer, P. (Spring 1990). Clinical medical ethics. *The Journal of Clinical Ethics, 1*(1), 5-9.

Singer, P., Sieger, M., and Pellegrino, E. (Summer 1990). Research in clinical ethics. *The Journal of Clinical Ethics, 1*(2), 95-99.

Tubbs, J. (1990). *Recent theological approaches in medical ethics.* Unpublished doctoral dissertation, University of Virginia.

Chapter 6

Arnason, W. (1991). Directed donation: The relevance of race. *Hastings Center Report, 21*(6), 13-19.

Callahan, Daniel. (1987). *Setting Limits.* New York: Simon and Schuster.

Callahan, Daniel. (1990). *What Kind of Life.* New York: Simon and Schuster.

Callahan, Daniel. (1993). *That Troubled Dream of Life.* New York: Simon and Schuster.

Dowie, M. (1988). *We Have a Donor: The Bold New World of Organ Transplanting.* New York: St. Martin's.

Edinger, W. (1990). Respect for donor choice and the Uniform Anatomical Gift Act. *Journal of Medical Humanities, 11* (Fall), 135-142.

Fox, R. and Swazey, J. (1992). *Spare Parts: Organ Replacement in American Society.* New York: Oxford University Press.

Gift of Life Agency: Transplantation Society of Michigan. (July 1, 2001). Michigan Statistics. Ann Arbor, Michigan.

Lyon, J. (1986). Organ Transplants. *Second Opinion, 1,* 40-65.

Marty, M. (1990). *Healthy People 2000: A Role for America's Religious Communities.* Chicago: The Carter and Park Ridge Centers.

Prottas, J. and Battein, H. (1991). The willingness to give: The public and the supply of transplantable organs. *Journal of Health Politics, Policy and Law, 16,* 121-134.

Chapter 7

Annas, G. (1994). The empire of death: How culture and economics affect informed consent in the U.S., the U.K., and Japan. *American Journal of Law and Medicine, 20*(4), 357-394.

Aycock, D. (1996). Of gourmet chefs and short-order cooks: Speculations on Worthington's speculations. *Journal of Psychology and Christianity, 15,* 223-227.

Davis, K., Collins, K., Schoen, C., and Morris, C. (1995). Choice Matters. *Health Affairs, 14*(2), 99-112.

Etheredge, L., Jones, S., Lewin, L. (1996). Marketwatch. *Health Affairs, 15*(4), 93-104.

Hogue, K. (2001). Chair, Council on Psychiatry and Law of American Psychiatric Association.

Hungate, R. (1996). Whither quality? *Health Affairs, 15*(4), 11.

Kohlberg, L. (1981). *Essays on Moral Development.* San Francisco: Harper and Row.

Lewin, M. and Jones, S. (1996). The market comes to Medicare. *Health Affairs, 15*(4), 57-61.

Luft, H. (1996). Modifying Managed Competition. *Health Affairs, 15*(1), 23-38.

Miller, F. (1996). Foreword: The promise and problem of capitation. *American Journal of Law, 22*(2-3), 167-172.

Morreim, E. (1995). Lifestyles of the risky and infamous: From managed care to managed lives. *Hastings Center Report, 25*(November-December), 5-12.

Pellegrino, E. (1994a). Allocation of resources at the bedside: The intersections of economics law, and ethics. *Kennedy Institute of Ethics Journal, 4*(4), 309-317.

Pellegrino, E. (1994b). Managed care and managed competition: Some ethical reflections. *Calyx Ethical Issues in Paediatrics, 4*(4), 1-5.

Rest, J. (1999). *Post-Conventional Moral Thinking: A Neo-Kohlbergian Approach.* Hillsdale, NJ: Erlbaum.

Rodwin, M. (1993), *Medicine, Money and Morals.* New York: Oxford University Press.

Sharfstein, S. (1995). Mental Disorder, Morals, and Money. *Health Affairs, 14*(3), 277-278.

Shenitz, B. (1992). "Patients left out in the cold." *Newsweek,* November 23, 1992, p. 48.

Walker, B. (1992). *USA Today.* Editorial: Self-insured firms' health benefits at risk. November 11, p. 12A.

Wells, K. (1995). Care for depression in a changing environment. *Health Affairs, 14,* 78-89.

Worthington, E. (1996). Speculations about new directions in helping marriages and families that arise from pressures of managed mental health care. *Journal of Psychology and Christianity, 15,* 197-212.

Chapter 8

Anderson, G. (1999). Nondirectiveness in prenatal genetics. *Nursing Ethics, 6*(2), 126-136.

Blank, R. H. (1989). Human genetic intervention: Portent of a brave new world? *Journal of Interdisciplinary Studies, 1*(1-2), 103-121.

Caskey, C. Thomas. (1991). The Genome Project and clinical medicine. Conference on legal and ethical issues raised by the Human Genome Project. Houston, March 7.

Clinton, W. (1993). *The President's Health Security Plan.* New York: Time Books.

Davis, B.D. (1990). The human genome and other initiatives. *Science, 249*(July), 342-343.

Duster, T. (1990). *Backdoor to Eugenics.* New York: Routledge.

Fletcher, John C. (1991). Religious communities and genetic research. Conference on Genetics and a Human Future. Valparaiso, IN, March 1991.

Gaylin, W. (2000). Nondirective counseling or advice. *Hastings Center Report, 30* (3), 31-33.

McGee, G. (1997). *The Perfect Baby.* New York: Rowman.

Nelson, J. Robert. (1994). *On the new frontiers of genetics and religion.* Grand Rapids, MI: Wm. B. Eerdmans Publishing Co.

Singer, P. (1991). Review essay. *Bioethics, 5*(3), 257-264.

Watson, J.D. (1990). The human genome project: Past, present, and future. *Science, 248,* 44.

Wertz, D.C. and Fletcher, J.C. (1989). *Ethics and Human Genetics: A Cross-Cultural Perspective.* New York: Springer-Verlag.

Chapter 9

Barbour, I. (1993). *Ethics in an Age of Technology.* San Francisco: Harper.

Bronzino, J.D., Smith, V.H., and Wade, M.L. (1990). *Medical Technology and Society.* New York: McGraw-Hill.

Callahan, D. (1993). *The Troubled Dream of Life: Living with Mortality.* New York: Simon and Schuster.

Davis, A.B. (1981). *Medicine and Its Technology: An Introduction to the History of Medical Instrumentation.* Westport, CT: Greenwood Press.

di Norcia, V. (1994). Ethics, technology development, and innovation. *Business Ethics Quarterly, 4*(3), 235-252.

Finkelstein, J.L., (1990). Biomedicine and technocratic power. *Hastings Center Report, 2,* 13-16.

Howell, J.D., ed. (1988). *Technology and American Medical Practice 1880-1930: An Anthology of Sources.* New York: Garland.

Office of Technology Assessment. Congress of the United States. (1978).

Reiser, S.J. (1978). *Medicine and the Reign of Technology.* Cambridge: Cambridge University Press.

Reiser, S.J. and Anbar, M., eds. (1984). *The Machine at the Bedside: Strategies for Using Technology in Patient Care.* Cambridge: Cambridge University Press.

Relman, A. (1979). Technology costs and evalutation. *New England Journal of Medicine. 301*(December 27), 1444-1445.

Thomas, L. (1974). The future impact of science and technology on medicine. *Bio Science 24*(2), 99-105; reprinted in Hickman, L. 1981. *Technology and Human Affairs.* St. Louis: Mosby.

Bibliography of Bioethics, 1975-2000

Audrey Davis (1981, p. 245) notes that "The only specific bibliography on surgical instruments was prepared by Anne Honor Clulow, *A Bibliography of the Litera-*

ture on Surgical Instruments, 1875-1900. London: Diploma in Librarianship Thesis, May 1961, in the University Library."

Cowan, R., ed., (1993). Biomedical and behavioral technology. *Technology and Culture, 34*(4).

Erlen, J. (1984). *The History of the Health Care Sciences and Health Care, 1700-1980: A Selective Annotated Bibliography.* New York: Garland.

Index catalogue of the Surgeon-General's Office of the U.S. Army.

Index Medicus.

Chapter 10

Beauchamp, T. and Childress, J. (1994). *Principles of Biomedical Ethics.* New York: Oxford.

Brody, H. (1981). *Ethical Decisions in Medicine.* Boston: Little, Brown.

Browning, D. (1980). *Pluralism and Personality: William James and Some Contemporary Cultures of Psychology.* Lewisburg, PA: Bucknell University Press.

Butler, R.N. (1975). *Why Survive?* New York: Harper.

Childress, J.F. (1997). *Practical Reasoning in Bioethics.* Bloomington, IN: Indiana University Press.

Davis, A. and Aroskar, M. (1997). *Ethical Dilemmas and Nursing.* Stamford, CT: Appleton.

Donagan, A. (1977). *The Theory of Morality.* Chicago: The University of Chicago Press.

Foley, J. (1981). Lecture presented to Summer Institutes on Old Age at Case Western Reserve University in Cleveland, Ohio. Funded by National Endowment for the Humanities.

Fowler, J. (1981). *Stages of Faith.* San Franciso: Harper.

Fowler, J. and Keen, S. (1978). *Life-Maps.* Minneapolis: Winston Press.

Fry, S. and Veatch, R. (2000). *Case Studies in Nursing Ethics,* Second Edition. Sudbury, MA: Jones and Bartlett Publishers.

Gadow, S. (1980). Medicine, ethics, and the elderly. *The Gerontologist, 20*(6), 680-685.

Gewirth, A. (1982). *Human Rights: Essays on Justification and Applications.* Chicago: The University of Chicago Press.

Gutmann, D. (1980). Observations on culture and mental health in later life. In *Handbook of Mental Health and Aging.* (pp. 429-447). Englewood Cliffs, NJ: Prentice-Hall.

James, W. (1909). *A Pluralistic Universe.* New York: Longmans, Green and Co.

James, W. (1911). *Some Problems of Philosophy.* New York: Longmans, Green and Co.

James, W. (1950). *The Principles of Psychology.* 2 vols. New York: Dover Publications, Inc. Original Publication 1890.

Katz, J., Capron, A.M., and Glass, E.S. eds. (1972). *Experimentation with Human Beings: The Authority of the Investigator, Subject, Professions, and State in the Human Experimentation Process.* New York: Russell Sage Foundation.

Kegan, R. (1982). *The Evolving Self.* Cambridge: Harvard University Press.

Kohlberg, L. (1973). Stages and aging in moral development: Some speculations. *Gerontologist, 13,* 497-502.

Kohlberg, L. (1974). Education, moral development and faith. *Journal of Moral Education, 4,* 5-16.

Kohlberg, L. (1981). *The Philosophy of Moral Development: Moral Stages and the Idea of Justice, Vol. 1. Essays on Moral Development.* San Francisco: Harper and Row.

Lasch, D. (1978). *The Culture of Narcissism: American Life in an Age of Diminishing Expectations.* New York: W.W. Norton and Company.

Levinson, H. (1978). *Science, Metaphysics, and the Chance of Salvation: An Interpretation of the Thought of William James.* Missoula, MT: Scholars Press.

Loewy, E. (1996). *The Textbook of Health Care Ethics.* New York: Plenum.

Outka, G. (1972). *Agape: An Ethical Analysis.* New Haven, CT: Yale University Press.

Outka, G. and Redder, J.P. Jr., eds. (1993). *Prospects for a Common Morality.* Princeton, NJ: Princeton University Press.

Ratzan, R.M. (1980). Being old makes you different. *Hastings Center Report,10*(5) 32.

Ratzan, R.M. (1981). The experiment that wasn't. *The Gerentologist, 21*(3), 297-302.

Sarton, M. (1973). *As We Are Now.* New York: Norton.

Spooner, W. (1914). The Golden Rule. In J. Hastings (Ed.), *Encyclopedia of Religion and Ethics,* Volume 6, pp. 310-312. New York: Charles Scribners.

Van Tassel, D. Editor. (1979). *Aging, Death, and the Completion of Being.* Philadelphia: University of Pennsylvania Press.

Veatch, R., ed. (1979). *Life Span.* New York: HarperCollins.

Wallwork, E. (1980). Morality, religion, and Kohlberg's theory. In B. Munsey (Ed.), *Moral Development, Moral Education, and Kohlberg.* Birmingham, AL: Religious Education Press.

Chapter 11

Adorno, T.W., Frenkel-Brunswik, E., and Levinson, D. (1950). *The Authoritarian Personality.* New York: Harper and Row.

Associated Press. (1996). "Religion question headed to appeals court (in Detroit)." *The Pioneer,* February 10. Big Rapids, Michigan. p. 2.

Astin, J.A. et al. (2000). The efficacy of "distant healing": A systematic review of randomized trials. *Annals of Internal Medicine.*

Callahan, S. (1999). A new synthesis. *Second Opinion, 1*(September) 57-78.

Campbell, C. (1999). Liberty and death in Oregon. *The Christian Century,* May 5, 498-500.

Carroll, J. and Wilson, R. (1980). *Too Many Pastors.* New York: The Pilgrim Press.

Chang, P. and Bompadre, V. (1999). Crowded pulpits: Observations and explanations of the clergy oversupply in the Protestant churches, 1950-1993. *Journal for the Scientific Study of Religion. 38* (3), 398-410.

Colston, L.G. and Johnson, P.E. (1972). *Personality and Christian Faith.* Nashville: Abingdon.

DeVries, R. and Subedi, J. (1998). *Bioethics and Society: Constructing the Ethical Enterprise.* Upper Saddle River, NJ: Prentice-Hall.

Douglas, W.G.T. (1957). *Predicting Ministerial Effectiveness.* Unpublished PhD dissertation. Cambridge, MA: Harvard University.

Fox, R. (1994). The entry of the U.S. bioethics into the 1990s. In *A Matter of Principles.* (pp. 21-71). Valley Forge, PA: Trinity Press International.

Hanford, J.T. (1974). *A Review and Critique of Methodology in the History of Psychology of Religion 1880-1960: Searching for a Synopsis.* Unpublished ThD dissertation. Denver, CO: Iliff School of Theology.

Hauerwas, S. (1994). *Dispatches from the Front: Theological Engagements with the Secular.* Durham, NC: Duke University Press.

Hiltner, S. and Colston, L. (1961). *The Context of Pastoral Counseling.* Nashville, TN: Abingdon.

Hofstadter, R. (1963). *Anti-intellectualism in American Life.* New York: Knopf.

James, W. (1902, 1961). *The Varieties of Religious Experience.* New York: Collier Books.

Koenig, H. (1994). *Aging and God.* Binghamton, NY: The Haworth Press.

Koenig, H. (1997). *Is Religion Good for Your Health.* Binghamton, NY: The Haworth Press.

Koenig, H. (1999). *The Healing Power of Faith.* New York: Simon & Schuster.

Koenig, H., Lamar, T., and Lamar, B. (1997). *A Gospel for the Mature Years.* Binghamton, NY: The Haworth Press.

Koenig, H. McCullough, M., and Larson, D. (2001). *Handbook of Religion and Health.* New York: Oxford University Press.

Koenig, H. and Weaver, A. (1997). *Counseling Troubled Older Adults.* Nashville, TN: Abingdon.

Marsden, G. (1997). *The Outrageous Idea of Christian Scholarship.* New York: Oxford University Press.

Menges, R.J. and Dittes, J.E. (1965). *Psychological Studies of Clergymen: Abstracts of Research.* New York: Thomas Nelson and Sons.

Noll, M. (1994). *The Scandal of the Evangelical Mind.* Grand Rapids, MI: Eerdmans.

Religious News Service. (1996). "YDS opt to fight laxity." *The Christian Century.* January 17, p. 39.

Rokeach, M. (1960). *The Open and Closed Mind.* New York: Basic Books.

Rokeach, M. (1964). *The Three Christs of Ypsilanti.* New York: Knopf.

Rokeach, M. (1968). *Beliefs, Attitudes, and Values.* San Francisco: Jossey-Bass.

Rokeach, M. (1969). Value systems in religion. *Review of Religious Research, 11:* 3-39.

Rokeach, M. (1970). Commentary on the commentaries. *Review of Religious Research, 11:* 155-162.

The SUPPORT Principal Investigators. (1995). A controlled trial to improve care for seriously ill hospitalized patients. *Journal of the American Medical Association, 274*(20), 1591-1598.

Young, D. (1996). Assisted suicide and the sacred. *Grand Rapids Press,* September 22, pp. E1, E4.

Chapter 12

American Association of Managed Care Nurses. (2000). *A Nurse's Introduction to Managed Care.* Glen Allen, VA: American Association of Managed Care Nurses.

Duckett, L. and Ryden, M. (1994). Education for ethical nursing practice. In J. Rest and D. Narvaez (Eds.), *Moral Development in the Professions,* (pp. 51-70). Hillsdale, NJ: Erlbaum.

Freidson, E. (1990). The centrality of professionalism to health care. *Jurimetrics Journal, 30* (Summer), 431-445.

NursingInsider. (May 5, 2000). Nyack Nurses Win. <http://NursingWorld.org>. American Nurses Association.

Rest, J. (1994). *Moral Development in the Professions.* Hillsdale, NJ: Erlbaum.

Rest, J. (1998). Post-Conventional Moral Thinking. Minnesota: Draft of Manuscript for Publication, May 23.

Rest, J. (1999). *Post-Conventional Moral Thinking: A Neo-Kohlbergian Approach.* Hillsdale, NJ: Erlbaum.

Sheehan, T.J., Husted, S.D., Candee, D., Cook, C.D., and Bargen, M. (1980). Moral judgment as a predictor of clinical performance. *Evaluation and the Health Professions, 3*(4), 393-404.

Shelly, J. and Miller, A. (1999). *Called to Care.* Illinois: InterVarsity Press.

Conclusion

American Hospital Association. (1972). Patient's Bill of Rights.

Levine, C. (1997). Postscript: Should doctors be able to refuse demands for "futile" treatment? In C. Levine (Ed.), *Taking Sides: Clashing Views on Controversial Bioethical Issues,* Seventh Edition (p. 131). Guilford, CT: The Dushkin Publishing Group.

The SUPPORT Principal Investigators. (1995). *Journal of the American Medical Association, 274*(20), 1591-1598.

Index

Adkins, Janet and Ron, 111
Ageism, 93
Aging. *See also* Elderly
  biomedical ethics course, 91-102
  as gift, 45
  and life cycle perspective, 89-91
  and narcissism, 86-87
Alternative medicine, 113
American Medical Association (AMA),
  3, 114, 120
  power of, 77
American Nurses Association (ANA),
  122, 123, 124
Anderson, Gwen, 71, 120
Anti-intellectualism, and religion, 104
Aroskar, Milo, 100
Artificial organ technology, 54
Astin, John, 114
Augustine, St., 95
Autonomy, 10, 94
Avery, William, 37

Barbour, Ian, 80, 81
Barth, Karl, 36
Becoming Adult, Becoming Christian,
  32, 33, 36
Beliefs, and motivation, 15
Beneficence, 10, 94
Bible, in Fowler's work, 29, 33, 34-35
Bioethics
  emergence of, 3
  religion in, 6, 46-47
  secularization of, 4
  term, 2
  therapeutic approach to, 41, 43
Biomedical ethics
  GGP funds for, 67
  and medical technology, 78
Biomedical ethics and aging course
  assignments, 99-100

Biomedical ethics and aging course
  (continued)
  case studies, 97-99
  description, 91-92
  evaluation, 101-102
  introduction to, 92-93
  outline, 93
  principles, 94-95
Blank, Robert, 67
Blood pressure measurement, 75-76
Bompadre, Viviana, 106
Bouma, Hessel, 70
Brody, Howard, 99
Browning, Donald, 86, 87
Butler, R., 92, 100

C-SPAN, health care issues, 64, 65
Callahan, Daniel, 4, 5, 55, 79
Callahan, Sidney, 113
Campus ministry, 103, 104
Caring, 43
Carroll, Jackson, 106
Caskey, Thomas, 69, 70
Celera Genomics, 71
Chandler School of Theology, 27
Chang, Patricia, 106
Children's Health Insurance Program
  (CHIP), 65
Childress, James, 96, 99
Christian faith
  and care, 129-130
  evangelical vs. liberal, 37
  and faith development theory, 29,
    31, 39
  Fowler on, 36
Christian Scientists, 6
Christian standard of care, 59
Christian therapy, 41, 44
Civil disobedience, 9

THE HAWORTH PASTORAL PRESS
Pastoral Care, Ministry, and Spirituality
Richard Dayringer, ThD
Senior Editor

LIFE CYCLE: PSYCHOLOGICAL AND THEOLOGICAL PERCEPTIONS by Richard Dayringer. "This is a terrific book. Dayringer takes us back to childhood and moves us through time, providing fresh new insights into each stage of life." *Harold G. Koenig, MD, Associate Professor of Medicine and Psychiatry, Duke University Medical Center, Durham, NC*

A THEOLOGY FOR PASTORAL PSYCHOTHERAPY: GOD'S PLAY IN SACRED SPACES by Brian W. Grant. "A compassionate and sophisticated synthesis of theology and psychoanalysis. Grant's wise, warm grasp binds a community of healers with the personal qualities, responsibilities, and burdens of the pastoral psychotherapist." *David E. Scharff, MD, Co-Director, International Institute of Object Relations Therapy*

LOSSES IN LATER LIFE: A NEW WAY OF WALKING WITH GOD, SECOND EDITION by R. Scott Sullender. "Continues to be a timely and helpful book. There is an empathetic tone throughout, even though the book is a bold challenge to grieve for the sake of growth and maturity and faithfulness. . . . An important book." *Herbert Anderson, PhD, Professor of Pastoral Theology, Catholic Theological Union, Chicago, Illinois*

CARING FOR PEOPLE FROM BIRTH TO DEATH edited by James E. Hightower Jr. "An expertly detailed account of the hopes and hazards folks experience at each stage of their lives. Your empathy will be deepened and your care of people will be highly informed." *Wayne E. Oates, PhD, Professor of Psychiatry Emeritus, School of Medicine, University of Louisville, Kentucky*

HIDDEN ADDICTIONS: A PASTORAL RESPONSE TO THE ABUSE OF LEGAL DRUGS by Bridget Clare McKeever. "This text is a must-read for physicians, pastors, nurses, and counselors. It should be required reading in every seminary and Clinical Pastoral Education program." *Martin C. Helldorfer, DMin, Vice President, Mission, Leadership Development and Corporate Culture, Catholic Health Initiatives—Eastern Region, Pennsylvania*

THE EIGHT MASKS OF MEN: A PRACTICAL GUIDE IN SPIRITUAL GROWTH FOR MEN OF THE CHRISTIAN FAITH by Frederick G. Grosse. "Thoroughly grounded in traditional Christian spirituality and thoughtfully aware of the needs of men in our culture. . . . Close attention could make men's groups once again a vital spiritual force in the church." *Eric O. Springsted, PhD, Chaplain and Professor of Philosophy and Religion, Illinois College, Jacksonville, Illinois*

THE HEART OF PASTORAL COUNSELING: HEALING THROUGH RELATIONSHIP, REVISED EDITION by Richard Dayringer. "Richard Dayringer's revised edition of *The Heart of Pastoral Counseling* is a book for every person's pastor and a pastor's every person." *Glen W. Davidson, Professor, New Mexico Highlands University, Las Vegas, New Mexico*

WHEN LIFE MEETS DEATH: STORIES OF DEATH AND DYING, TRUTH AND COURAGE by Thomas W. Shane. "A kaleidoscope of compassionate, artfully tendered pastoral encounters that evoke in the reader a full range of emotions." *The Rev. Dr. James M. Harper, III, Corporate Director of Clinical Pastoral Education, Health Midwest; Director of Pastoral Care, Baptist Medical Center and Research Medical Center, Kansas City Missouri*

A MEMOIR OF A PASTORAL COUNSELING PRACTICE by Robert L. Menz. "Challenges the reader's belief system. A humorous and abstract book that begs to be read again, and even again." *Richard Dayringer, ThD, Professor and Director, Program in Psychosocial Care, Department of Medical Humanities; Professor and Chief, Division of Behavioral Science, Department of Family and Community Medicine, Southern Illinois University School of Medicine*

Order Your Own Copy of
This Important Book for Your Personal Library!

BIOETHICS FROM A FAITH PERSPECTIVE
Ethics in Health Care for the Twenty-First Century

_____in hardbound at $49.95 (ISBN: 0-7890-1509-9)
_____in softbound at $19.95 (ISBN: 0-7890-1510-2)

COST OF BOOKS_____

OUTSIDE USA/CANADA/
MEXICO: ADD 20%____

POSTAGE & HANDLING_____
*(US: $4.00 for first book & $1.50
for each additional book)
Outside US: $5.00 for first book
& $2.00 for each additional book)*

SUBTOTAL_____

in Canada: add 7% GST____

STATE TAX____
*(NY, OH & MIN residents, please
add appropriate local sales tax)*

FINAL TOTAL____
*(If paying in Canadian funds,
convert using the current
exchange rate, UNESCO
coupons welcome.)*

❏ **BILL ME LATER:** ($5 service charge will be added)
(Bill-me option is good on US/Canada/Mexico orders only;
not good to jobbers, wholesalers, or subscription agencies.)

❏ Check here if billing address is different from
shipping address and attach purchase order and
billing address information.

Signature_____

❏ **PAYMENT ENCLOSED: $_____**

❏ **PLEASE CHARGE TO MY CREDIT CARD.**

❏ Visa ❏ MasterCard ❏ AmEx ❏ Discover
❏ Diner's Club ❏ Eurocard ❏ JCB

Account # _____

Exp. Date_____

Signature_____

Prices in US dollars and subject to change without notice.

NAME_____

INSTITUTION_____

ADDRESS_____

CITY_____

STATE/ZIP_____

COUNTRY_____ COUNTY (NY residents only)_____

TEL_____ FAX_____

E-MAIL_____

May we use your e-mail address for confirmations and other types of information? ❏ Yes ❏ No
We appreciate receiving your e-mail address and fax number. Haworth would like to e-mail or fax special
discount offers to you, as a preferred customer. **We will never share, rent, or exchange your e-mail address
or fax number.** We regard such actions as an invasion of your privacy.

Order From Your Local Bookstore or Directly From
The Haworth Press, Inc.
10 Alice Street, Binghamton, New York 13904-1580 • USA
TELEPHONE: 1-800-HAWORTH (1-800-429-6784) / Outside US/Canada: (607) 722-5857
FAX: 1-800-895-0582 / Outside US/Canada: (607) 722-6362
E-mail: getinfo@haworthpressinc.com
PLEASE PHOTOCOPY THIS FORM FOR YOUR PERSONAL USE.
www.HaworthPress.com